DIAGNOSTIC ERRORS IN TRAUMA CARE

and how to avoid them

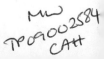

This book is dedicated to all the patients, the world over, whose missed injuries form the clinical experience and basis for this book

DIAGNOSTIC ERRORS IN TRAUMA CARE

and how to avoid them

by

H.R. Guly MBBS, MRCP (UK)

Consultant in Accident and Emergency,
Derriford Hospital, Plymouth.
Honorary Civilian Consultant
in Accident and Emergency to the Royal Navy

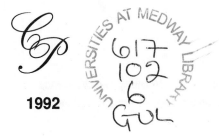

1992

Published by Clinical Press Limited,
Redland Green Farm, Redland Green, Redland, Bristol, BS6 6HF

ISBN: 1 85457 027 7

Printed in Great Britain by Antony Rowe Ltd
Typesetting by The Devonshire Press, Torquay, Devon.

Contents

Introduction

For a variety of reasons to be explored in this book, it is common for doctors to make diagnostic errors when managing injured patients. While it is impossible to avoid all mistakes, even avoidable ones, doctors should always search out their mistakes and learn from them (McIntyre and Popper, 1983). By bringing together the experience of an accident and emergency (A&E) consultant who has a large experience of sorting out the diagnostic errors made by his junior staff (and, on occasion, by himself!) and the published literature on the subject, my hope is that doctors may be able to learn from the mistakes of others and thus make fewer of their own, thereby improving patient care. (In my opinion, the emphasis on the importance of making a correct diagnosis should be that it will improve patient care and not that it will avoid the legal consequences of an error.)

Although this book concentrates on diagnostic errors, it must not be forgotten that other aspects of A & E work, such as patient management and doctor–patient communication, can also be improved. Many of the reasons explored in this book as causes for misdiagnosis will also be related to other problems in A & E departments.

This book is therefore aimed at doctors working at the sharp end: A & E and orthopaedic junior medical staff and general practitioners, especially those who work in A & E departments. A & E consultants will, I hope, find it useful, and I hope it will provide teaching material and can be used as a basis for future research on the subject. In addition, I hope that sections of it may be useful for other doctors who treat injured patients and for managers who are responsible for providing A & E services and for answering complaints against A & E departments.

It must be remembered that policies on X-rays vary from hospital to hospital. In one hospital a doctor requesting foot X-rays will be given an AP and an oblique X-ray to interpret, whereas in another hospital he may be given a lateral X-ray of the foot as well. This needs to be borne in mind when reading my advice on what X-rays to request. The management of injuries also varies from hospital to hospital. Clearly, in a hospital with a hand surgeon who repairs collateral ligament tears of the proximal interphalangeal joints, it is more important to diagnose these injuries than in a hospital where they are treated conservatively, possibly no differently from a sprain.

Lastly, this book is not a comprehensive list of things which can go wrong, as there can be no injury which has not been missed at some time by somebody for whatever reason. I have tried to include the commoner and more important missed diagnoses, but this book needs to be read in conjunction with an orthopaedic textbook, a radiological atlas of normal variants and individual A & E departmental guidelines on the management of specific injuries.

REFERENCE

McIntyre N. and Popper K. (1983) The critical attitude in medicine: the need for a new ethic. *Br. Med. J.,* **287,** 1919–23.

1 The importance of diagnosis

When a patient presents to a doctor, it has traditionally been taught that an accurate diagnosis is essential, and this is self-evident. However, it has been argued that, if a patient has a minor chest wall injury, his treatment will be the same whether or not there is a rib fracture and therefore X-rays to prove or disprove the presence of a rib fracture are unnecessary (de Lacey, 1976) and should not be done, particularly when a department has to work within a limited budget. Similar arguments have been advanced to suggest that X-rays are unnecessary for the management of toe injuries, many head injuries (Evans, 1977), nose injuries (de Lacey et al., 1977), injuries at the base of the fifth metatarsal (Dunlop et al., 1986) and other conditions. It has been argued, with some justification, that what matters is to recognize which patients will respond to different forms of treatment, rather than to argue over the truth of the diagnosis with which a patient's problem is labelled (McCartney, 1987).

This implies that patients come to a doctor only for treatment, whereas patients may come for many other reasons, including: wanting an explanation for their symptoms; a prognosis or just reassurance. Asher (1972) states that knowing the name of the disease that afflicts them makes patients feel that they have power over the disease, and there is no doubt that patients with a very limited knowledge of anatomy and none of pathology are happier when they 'know' what is wrong with them. Doctors should provide patients with the information they seek, and this usually includes a diagnosis. Diagnoses can be made at different levels and with different degrees of certainty, and how far one investigates a patient to reach a diagnosis will depend on what is acceptable in relation to the risks and benefits of investigation and therapeutic options (Hoffbrand, 1987). To this, some might add 'costs'. Simple radiological investigation usually carry negligible risks, except possibly during pregnancy.

Another reason for confirming a diagnosis radiologically is that the doctor's clinical diagnosis may be wrong (as this book will demonstrate). While it may be argued that there is no indication to X-ray a suspected fractured toe, as its treatment is the same as that for a bruised toe (assuming there is no wound), if the clinical diagnosis was wrong and a dislocated toe was missed, this might cause prolonged disability.

Finally, if a patient is discharged without being X-rayed and later consults another doctor who orders an X-ray which reveals a fracture, the patient is usually aggrieved and may lose confidence in the first doctor or hospital, even if the fracture did not require any specific treatment.

For these reasons, I will assume for the purposes of this book that it is important to make a correct diagnosis, even though it may not alter a patient's treatment, though I will try to distinguish between important and less important missed diagnoses.

WHAT INJURIES ARE MISSED AND HOW BIG IS THE PROBLEM?

These are obviously questions of vital importance, but they are very difficult and probably impossible to answer. Injured patients may be admitted or followed up by many different specialists and general practitioners and, if a diagnosis is made during follow-up, details may never get fed back to the doctor who made the original error. Some injuries may go undiagnosed for months or years (e.g. posterior dislocation of the shoulder) and other injuries (even serious ones, such as depressed skull fractures) may never be diagnosed if a patient suffers no complication and makes an uneventful recovery. One short study has tried to look at the total picture (Guly, 1984) but is almost certainly incomplete for the above reasons.

Other studies have looked at subgroups of injured patients. Some errors lead to complaints and medicolegal problems, and these have been looked at (see Tables 1.1, 1.2, 1.3). However, complainants are a very selected group and these errors, while clearly of great importance, are not necessarily representative of the whole problem.

Table 1.1 Trauma diagnostic errors in 250 cases of orthopaedic malpractice (Kellsey, 1975)

Central dislocation of hip (in multiple injuries)	2
Monteggia fracture	2
Fractured scaphoid	2
Arterial injury associated with leg fracture	2
Slipped upper femoral epiphysis	1
Fractured pubic ramus	1
Fractured femoral neck	1
Fracture-dislocation cervical spine	1
Compression fracture T1	1
Fracture-dislocation foot	1
Trans-scapho-perilunar dislocation	1

Table 1.2 Trauma missed or delayed diagnosis in 100 orthopaedic and accident cases considered by a medical defence organization (Thomas, 1986)

Foreign body	7
Nerve injury (open)	4
Lower cervical spine injury	3
Compartment syndrome	3
Bimalleolar fracture ankle	2
Fractured scaphoid	2
Slipped upper femoral epiphysis	2
Ruptured Achilles tendon	1

Table 1.3 Missed diagnoses reported to a medical defence organization in 1983
(Hawkins, 1985)

Missed fractures	
femur	11
scaphoid	10
rib	9
wrist	9
finger	9
lumbar vertebrae	8
tibia	8
fibula	7
hip	6
skull	5
radius	5
leg	5
ankle	5
neck	4
humerus	4
arm	4
pelvis	4
foot	4
clavicle	3
ulna	3
metacarpal	3
mandible	2
Foreign bodies	
glass	22
miscellaneous, e.g. metal/wood/bullet	27
in eye	7

The most common cause of a missed diagnosis is failure to interpret an X-ray properly (Chapter 3). The significant injuries missed on X-ray in one hospital over a year are shown in Table 1.4. Other published papers also have lists of significant injuries missed on X-ray over a shorter time (de Lacey et al., 1980; Carew-McColl, 1983; Guly, 1984).

Others have investigated failure to X-ray (Guly, 1986) (Chapter 2), multiple injuries (Chapter 22) and specific injuries, but there has been no large scale study on total missed injuries other than those missed on X-rays.

Table 1.4 Significant injuries missed on X-ray in patients who were discharged at one hospital in a year (Wardrope and Chennells, 1985)

Fractured scaphoid	11
Undisplaced greenstick fracture wrist	10
Fractured skull	10
Fractured zygoma	8
Blow out fracture	7
Fractured radial head	7
Fractured ribs	5
Fractured navicular	5
Wedge fracture spine	4
Fractured lateral malleolus	4
Fractured calcaneum	3
Fractured head of fibula	3
Fractured posterior malleolus	3
Fractured pubic ramus	3

Injuries of which 2 or fewer were missed are not included.

The answer to 'how big is the problem?' is therefore unknown. A significant percentage of injuries is missed because X-rays are misinterpreted. This varies from study to study but up to 30% of skull fractures may be missed (Chapter 6) and the incidence of missed cervical spine injuries may be higher (Chapter 7). Patients with uncommon injuries (e.g. dislocation of the lunate) or rare ones (e.g. fractured hook of hamate) stand a less than evens chance of having it diagnosed at presentation. Patients with multiple injuries have a high incidence of missed injuries, both minor and those contributing to mortality (Chapter 22).

The size of the problem is therefore significant.

FALSE POSITIVE DIAGNOSES

There are two types of diagnostic error: the missed diagnosis or false negative is when a significant injury is missed completely or is misdiagnosed as a more minor injury and the false positive is when a minor injury is misdiagnosed as a more serious one. False positive diagnoses are usually radiological diagnoses caused by a lack of knowledge of normal radiological anatomy such as epiphyses and nutrient arteries in long bones or by a lack of knowledge of normal variants such as bipartite bones, sesamoid and other accessory bones. Radiological artefacts, pre-existing diseases and old fractures and dislocations may also be diagnosed as acute injuries. Soft-tissue injuries may also be over-diagnosed, such as a longstanding ligamentous laxity masquerading as an acute ligamentous rupture and the over-diagnosed meniscal tear in the knee.

False positive diagnoses in the A & E department are not as important as false negative ones, as the patient will usually be referred to someone more senior who should correct the diagnosis. However, this may not always occur, as demonstrated by a case in which an accessory bone was thought to be a fracture of the medial malleolus and underwent internal fixation (Coral, 1986).

False positive diagnoses which are later corrected should not be dismissed as unimportant, as they cause additional work and expense to the hospital, inconvenience and possible expense to patients who may have unnecessary plasters, time off work and visits to hospital, and they may also delay physiotherapy for soft tissue injuries. Some patients, having once been told that they have a fracture, subsequently refuse to believe that there was no bony injury, and this hinders their rehabilitation. However, a degree of caution by inexperienced A & E doctors is essential, and a small percentage of false positive diagnoses may be a necessary price to prevent the disastrous false negative. In this book I have concentrated on false negative diagnoses, though I mention the common false positives.

REFERENCES

Asher R. (1972) Making sense in "Richard Asher Talking Sense", pub. Pitman Medical, pp. 20–41.

Carew-McColl M. (1983) Radiological interpretation in an Accident and Emergency Department. *Br. J. Clin. Pract.*, **37**, 375–7.

Coral A. (1986) Os subtibiale mistaken for a recent fracture. *Br. Med. J.*, **292**, 1571–2.

de Lacey G. (1976) Clinical and economic aspects of the use of X-rays in the Accident and Emergency Department. *Proc. R. Soc. Med.*, **69**, 758–9.

de Lacey G., Barker A., Harper J. et al. (1980) An assessment of the clinical effects of reporting Accident and Emergency Radiographs. *Br. J. Radiol.*, **53**, 304–9.

de Lacey G.J., Wignall B.K., Hussein S. et al. (1977) The radiology of nasal injuries: problems of interpretation and clinical relevance. *Br. J. Radiol.*, **50**, 412–4.

Dunlop M.G., Beattie T.F., White G.K. et al. (1986) Guidelines for selective radiological assessment of inversion ankle injuries. *Br. Med. J.*, **293**, 603–5.

Evans K.T. (1977) The Radiologists dilemma. *Br. J. Radiol.*, **50**, 299–301.

Guly H.R. (1984) Missed diagnoses in an Accident and Emergency Department. *Injury*, **15**, 403–6.

Guly H.R. (9186) Fractures not X-rayed. *Arch. Emerg. Med.*, **3**, 159–62.

Hawkins C. (1985) Perennial Pitfalls in "Mishap or Malpractice". Blackwell Scientific Publications, Oxford, pp. 130–154.

Hoffbrand B. (1987) Diagnosis and decisions – can we do better? *Postgrad. Med. J.*, **63**, 729–30.

Kellsey D.C. (1975) The anatomy of orthopaedic malpractice. *J. Bone Jt Surg.*, **57A**, 1013–18.

McCartney F.J. (1987) Diagnostic Logic. *Br. Med. J.*, **295**, 1325–31.

Thomas T.G. (1986) Orthopaedic manholes and rabbit holes: some thoughts on medical negligence. *J. R. Soc. Med.*, **79**, 701–7.

Wardrope J. and Chennells P.M. (1985) Should all casualty radiographs be reviewed? *Br. Med.J.*, **290**, 1638–40.

2   Errors in clinical diagnosis

THE DIAGNOSTIC PROCESS

The traditional approach to diagnosis is that the doctor takes a history, examines the relevant part and then the whole patient and, from his findings, makes a provisional diagnosis (or sometimes a differential diagnosis). Following investigations (usually X-rays in cases of trauma) to prove or disprove this provisional diagnosis, the final diagnosis is then made. Sometimes the final diagnosis can be made from clinical findings alone. Thus the traditional diagnostic process can be summarized as:

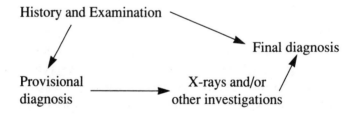

With much interest and research into computerized diagnosis, the way in which doctors reach a diagnosis has been looked at, and it is clear that in practice many diagnoses are reached in other ways (McCartney, 1987). However, even if a patient comes into an A & E department with an injury diagnosable by a casual glance, it is still necessary to go through a traditional approach in order to diagnose less obvious associated injuries or complications.

Errors in the final diagnosis may result from errors at any stage of this diagnostic process.

It must be stressed that every doctor who sees a patient who is new to him must approach that patient without preconceived ideas, as these inevitably alter the doctor/patient relationship and the approach to making a diagnosis.

If the patient has been seen by two previous doctors for the same problem and neither has found a significant cause, it is possible that the patient is over-reacting for whatever reason. It is also possible that the previous two doctors have both missed something. The Medical Defence Union's Annual Report of 1983 describes a patient with a comminuted fracture of her lower radius who was not X-rayed until her eighth visit to an A & E department.

An obvious hazard is the patient who is in police custody, as he may be approached without sympathy (which will make proper communication for obtaining a history impossible) or, worse, by assuming that he is 'swinging the lead'.

A less obvious problem is the nurse who asks, 'Will you see the patient with the sprained ankle in cubicle 8?' This may be the first step in a chain of errors, leading to a missed fractured calcaneum or ruptured Achilles tendon.

HISTORY

The history of the mechanism of injury and the forces involved is a very important first step in establishing a diagnosis and, while failure to take a history is rarely the only reason why a diagnosis is missed, it is frequently a major contributory factor, leading to failure to examine the relevant parts and wrong decisions as to who to X-ray.

Thus in a patient with an injured ankle: a history of a fall onto the heel suggests the possibility of a calcaneal fracture; an inversion injury commonly causes an injury to the lateral ligament or to one of the malleoli, and a sudden onset of pain behind the ankle occurring during exertion suggests an injury to the Achilles tendon. If a patient has a hand laceration caused by broken glass, there is likely to be a tendon or nerve injury and there is the possibility of a glass foreign body within the wound, whereas if the laceration has been caused by a blow from a blunt object, there is likely to be an underlying fracture.

10

The history of some conditions is so characteristic (e.g. the ruptured Achilles tendon or the pulled elbow) as to be almost diagnostic, and there are other conditions which may only be diagnosable by an accurate account of what happened, e.g. the dislocated patella which reduced spontaneously or the dislocated proximal interphalangeal joint of a finger which the patient pulled straight himself. This type of help will only be given if the patient is encouraged to say what happened, and will never be obtained by asking questions demanding a 'yes' or 'no' answer. This good communication will never occur if the patient senses the doctor to be antagonistic.

The history may also help to avoid a false positive diagnosis. For example, if a knee injury was caused by a direct blow, or if the patient with the injury was able to finish his game of football, then, whatever the findings on examination, there is not a recent meniscus injury.

Past Medical History

A knowledge of previous injuries may be of great relevance in establishing a diagnosis. Healing fractures may refracture, a history of previous knee problems might suggest a meniscus tear and an old skull fracture may be confused for a new injury. Medical conditions, such as malignancy or steroid therapy, may predispose to pathological fractures and so lower the threshold for requesting X-rays. Rigid spines due to ankylosing spondylitis may fracture with minimal trauma (Chapter 7) and anticoagulant therapy will predispose to bleeding, including intracranial haematoma. Many other conditions will also predispose to specific injuries, and so all patients with other than trivial injuries should have a medical history taken. Leaman found that taking an extended history from walking wounded patients directly influenced the management (not just the diagnosis) of 12% of them (Leaman, 1986).

It may be impossible to obtain a history from some patients, e.g. if comatose, confused, drunk, mentally handicapped, severely psychiatrically ill or if very young. Language difficulties may necessitate taking a history through an interpreter, which is never easy, and fractured mandibles and shortness of breath also cause communication difficulties.

This inability to obtain a history causes great diagnostic difficulty including, at worst, failure to realise that the patient has had an injury. Thus head injured patients may be diagnosed as being drunk or as having suffered a stroke (Galbraith, 1976), patients with fractured necks of femur will be assumed to have a flare up of osteo-arthritis (Eastwood, 1987), spinal injury may be diagnosed as torticollis (Guly, 1986) and an epiphyseal fracture of the terminal phalanx as a paronychia (Guly, 1986).

If a patient is unable to give a history, it is essential to try to obtain an eye-witness account of what happened. The history of a road accident should never just read 'RTA' as the mechanism of the injury and the type of impact may give clues as to the type of injuries expected. Ambulancemen should be prevented from leaving the A & E department until they have given this information. It is also important to enquire how a patient's condition has changed since he was first seen, as many an extradural haematoma has been missed or its diagnosis has been delayed by assuming that an unconscious patient has been in that state ever since the accident, whereas the information that the patient was talking and then became unconscious was available had anyone asked.

Lastly, it must not be forgotten that some people deliberately lie about their children's injuries (e.g. in child abuse) or their own injuries. It is impossible to know how often patients lie about their own injuries, but it is probably not rare and it usually occurs because of embarrassment about the circumstances of the injury, rather than for any gain. An obvious example is the patient with a laceration of the knuckle which it is claimed has an innocent cause, but which was, in fact, a punching injury sustained on an opponent's teeth. It is not, therefore, a simple wound to be sutured but is a dirty human bite injury, possibly compound into the metacarpophalangeal joint, and thus a serious injury. The wife who has been beaten up by her husband, but who claims to have fallen downstairs, is another example.

While the patient who has been misdiagnosed and mistreated as a result of giving a false history would have very little ground for complaint, one should still aim for a correct diagnosis, despite the patient's stupidity. If the findings on physical examination do not correspond with the history, the patient should be further pressed about what happened.

Practical points

● An understanding of the mechanism of injury and of what happened to the patient immediately afterwards is vital in establishing a diagnosis. Particular care should be exercised when this information cannot be obtained, as injuries are very likely to be missed in these circumstances.
● The past medical history may give very valuable clues to the diagnosis and may considerably influence the management of the patient.

EXAMINATION

It should go without saying that doctors must always examine the patient fully, but it has long been recognised that this does not always happen. Sir Zachary Cope (on abdominal pain) states:

"More harm is done because you do not look
Than from not knowing what is in the book." (Cope, 1972)

and Flatt (1979) on hand injuries, is even more sure:

"Errors in diagnosis can occur only because of errors
of omission and commission in the examination."

Soft tissue injuries of tendon, muscle, nerve and some ligaments can only be diagnosed clinically (though some of the latter may be confirmed by stress X-rays) and arterial injuries too should be diagnosed clinically, though they may need confirmation by angiography. If a proper clinical examination is not done, these injuries will be, and are, missed (Chapters 18 and 19).

Bony injuries will usually be diagnosed by X-rays, but it is essential that these are preceded by a clinical diagnosis based on a full and accurate clinical examination, as on this will depend which X-rays are requested and how they are interpreted. If a patient presents with an injured shoulder, to request just a 'shoulder X-ray' is valueless, as a supine AP shoulder X-ray may fail to demonstrate a posterior dislocation, an acromioclavicular or sternoclavicular dislocation or a fractured scapula, each of which may need specific X-rays to demonstrate it.

Diagnostic errors resulting from inadequate examination may occur for several reasons.

Firstly, doctors may not know how to examine for specific injuries. In my experience, most doctors starting a first job in an A & E department have only the vaguest idea about how to examine the musculoskeletal system and, in particular, seem unable to test for tendon injuries. This may have been learnt once but forgotten, although musculoskeletal diseases seem to have a low priority in a crowded medical school curriculum and I suspect that many doctors qualify without ever having been properly taught or tested on this. Even if a doctor can examine a patient, it may not be done for a variety of reasons. He may already have made a spot diagnosis and feel that a full examination is unnecessary. He may already have assessed the injury as minor or the patient as a malingerer or, if he is busy and there is a long wait for patients to be seen, he may deliberately be cutting corners to save time. Lastly, he may be working through an examination and, quite innocently, forget some aspect of it. It is essential that doctors develop a routine for examining joins, wounds, etc. and always stick to it.

One of the commonest omissions in examination which leads to missed diagnoses is the failure to examine the gait of patients with lower limb injuries (Guly, 1986). In a child with a greenstick fracture in the lower limb, it may be impossible to localise tenderness, and the only positive physical sign may be a refusal to weight bear. If a patient who has been diagnosed as having a minor leg injury refuses to weight bear or walks with a severe limp, the diagnosis should be reconsidered. (N.B. the ability to weight bear does not exclude a serious injury.)

It is recognized that pain from an injured part of the body may be referred distally. Thus neck problems may present with pain in the shoulder or elsewhere, and patients with hip problems may feel their pain in the thigh or the knee. This is especially true for slipped upper femoral epiphyses (Wilson, Jacobs and Schecter, 1965). Children with pulled elbow may localize their pain not only distally in the forearm or wrist, but occasionally it is felt proximally in the shoulder Illingworth, 1975). For this reason (and others), doctors examining an injured limb may wrongly localise the injury and examine and even X-ray the wrong part of the body (Guly, 1986). The examination of any joint should include an examination of the joints above and below it, especially if there is a discrepancy between symptoms and the findings on physical examination.

Lastly it needs to be recognized that a patient may have more than one injury (see Chapter 22) and so, although attention may be directed to the presenting injury, if a patient has been injured in a road accident or fall, the rest of the body should be briefly examined also. Even patients with a simple mechanism of injury may have more than one injury. Thus a patient with a Colles fracture may also have a fractured radial head (Cooney, Dobyns and Linscheid, 1980) and, even more commonly, an inversion injury to the ankle will cause not just an ankle injury but also a fracture of the base of the fifth metatarsal. This is another reason for examining the joint about and below any injury.

Patients are sometimes brought reluctantly to an A & E department by a friend or the ambulance service following an accident. If this has been a significant accident, they should be persuaded to be 'checked over' even if they argue that they are all right, as pain following an accident may have a delayed onset (Phillips and Baggoley, 1986) or they may be denying pain because they are more worried about a seriously injured relative. Pain usually starts within an hour, but it may be delayed for up to 9 hours (Melzack, Wall and Ty, 1982) and 22% of patients with soft tissue neck injuries may not develop pain for 12 hours (Deans, McGalliard and Rutherford, 1986).

Practical points

● Develop a systematic approach to physical examination and do a full examination every time. Once you are practised it takes little more time to do a full examination than to do a poor one.

● Method for examining a joint following trauma:

Look	position, deformity
	wounds, bruising, swelling scars, muscle wasting (suggest longstanding problems)
Feel	for deformity, swelling
	localize the point of maximum tenderness.
Move	examine the range of movement
	test for stability
Function	e.g. gait
Special tests	e.g. pulses and nerve function distal to a fracture

or tests for specific injuries, e.g. testing knee extension against gravity to exclude rupture of extensor mechanism

● Method for examining a wound following trauma:

Look at wound	type of wound
	size, shape, position
	edges — clean, incised or contused viable or non-viable
	depth
	appearance — age, contamination.

Exclude associated soft-tissue injury

Look distally	pulses and evidence of poor perfusion
	tendon function
	nerve function (motor/sensory)

Exclude underlying bone or joint injury — as above.

● Examine the joint above and the joint below the obvious injury

● Unless there is an obvious injury which clearly would contra-indicate it – always examine the gait of any patient with a lower limb injury

● When the department is busy, you may well be able to work faster but do not take short cuts. The patient would rather wait two hours and be treated properly than be out in half an hour and have something missed

PROVISIONAL DIAGNOSIS

Clearly if the history taking or physical examination has been inadequate, the provisional diagnosis will probably be wrong but, even if these have been done competently, errors will be made if the doctor does not think. Thus, if a heavy blow causes a laceration of the arm, it may also fracture an underlying bone. This fracture will be missed if the doctor merely notes the history and just sutures the wound without using the history he has obtained to make a provisional diagnosis. Time must be allowed to process the data the doctor has collected (Editorial, 1977).

Sometimes a doctor has never heard of a certain injury and does not know that such a condition exists. This makes it difficult to diagnose! Among recent casualty officers, less than a third had ever heard of a pulled elbow before starting to work in A & E (personal observations). There are other, usually uncommon, conditions which doctors may never have heard of, but many of these could be diagnosed at this stage with a bit of thought (but are often missed). Thus the patient who is unable actively to flex the distal interphalangeal joint of a finger following an injury in which he tried to resist an extension force, and yet who has got full passive movements, must have a ruptured flexor digitorum longus tendon to that finger even if the doctor has never heard of this (admittedly uncommon) condition.

Even if a patient clearly needs an X-ray, it is important that a provisional diagnosis is written down so that it can be compared with the X-ray findings. Only in this way, by testing his clinical diagnosis with the final diagnosis, will a doctor develop the experience and confidence he needs to make clinical diagnoses, which is a necessary skill for future general practitioners to acquire, as they will be expected to see and treat injured patients without easy access to X-rays.

If this provisional diagnosis differs significantly from the X-ray findings, it will be necessary to review the X-rays again (Chapter 4). This safeguard will occur if the notes read 'probable Colles fracture: XR-NBI', but will not if they read 'wrist injury: XR-NBI'.

Practical Points

- Use your loaf when you make your diagnosis.
- If your clinical method has been inadequate, you may make serious diagnostic errors and may be viewed as negligent.
- You may still make errors if your clinical methods are perfect but they will not be serious ones, and cannot be considered as negligent.

DECISION TO X-RAY

The decision to X-ray a patient to confirm or refute this provisional diagnosis will depend on the likelihood of finding a fracture, based on the clinical findings and the importance of the fracture. Thus it is important to have a much lower threshold for X-raying the cervical spine or the hip than for X-raying an uncomplicated chest wall injury, whose management will not be altered by finding a rib fracture.

Junior A & E doctors' clinical diagnoses of the presence or absence of a fracture are not very accurate. Thus patients thought to have no fractures on clinical grounds have been found to have radiological abnormalities in 6.1% (Morgan et al., 1980) and 8.7% (Warren and Fergusson, 1984) of cases, and X-rays taken for reassurance and for medico-legal reasons reveal 6% and 8% of unexpected abnormalities (de Lacey et al., 1979). Luckily these doctors also have a low threshold for requesting X-rays, and so fractures are not often missed in A & E departments because of failure to X-ray. The Royal College of Radiologists Working Party report (1985) found that only 0.03% of new patients in A & E departments had a limb fracture missed because it was not X-rayed at the initial visit.

The problem of fractures being missed because they were not X-rayed has been investigated (Guly, 1986). Of 31 fractures missed for this reason, in about half (including all the serious fractures) the decision not to X-ray was based on poor clinical method (e.g. failure to obtain a history of injury, failure to use this history in establishing the diagnosis, failure to localize the site of the injury, failure to examine the patient properly and overlooking an injury in a patient with more than one injury). The rest of the fractures were missed because the doctor felt that there was no fracture based on a good history and a good examination. None of these injuries was serious and some were very minor, and the decision not to request an X-ray would almost certainly not be called negligent (Holder, 1972).

Doctors who treat injured patients soon get experience of the common injuries and gain an impression as to which symptoms and signs or combinations of symptoms and signs point towards the presence or absence of a fracture. Unfortunately impressions may be mistaken, and it is important that these impressions are reinforced by facts. Several investigators have examined patients with head injuries and ankle injuries to draw up guidelines as to which patients require X-rays (Chapters 6 and 17) but unfortunately no guideline will pick up every fracture and, in the study of fractures not X-rayed discussed above (Guly, 1986), there were two skull fractures and four ankle and foot fractures, despite physical signs suggesting the absence of a fracture. More work needs to be done to draw up and validate guidelines as to who should be X-rayed although, even then, a few fractures will always be missed, but these should all be minor ones. Guidelines should only be guidelines and can never be absolute rules, and should never be used as a substitute for thought.

If any guideline is introduced, the reason for it should be made clear. The aim should be to assist doctors in making diagnostic decisions, thereby improving the care of an individual patient. On occasions, guidelines are introduced as a means of reducing X-ray examinations to save money (thereby assisting the community possibly, at a cost to the individual patient). If guidelines are introduced for these financial motives, the health authorities must accept legal and financial responsibilities for doctors in their employment if a fracture is missed and the guidelines are found unsatisfactory in court (Harvey and Roberts, 1987).

Occasionally injuries are missed because of a reluctance to X-ray a pregnant patient. The scatter from modern X-ray machines is minimal and, particularly if the patient has her abdomen covered with a lead apron, there is no contraindication to X-raying the skull/cervical spine/limbs, etc. X-rays of the lumbar spine and pelvis must expose the foetus to radiation, and clinical judgement must be made as to whether these parts are X-rayed, but if there is a reasonable chance of an injury the patient must be X-rayed, as to miss a significant injury will cause mother and foetus much more harm than will an X-ray.

REFERENCES

Cooney W.P., Dobyns J.H. & Linscheid R.L. (1980) Complications of Colles fracture. *J. Bone Jt Surg.*, **62A**, 613–9.

Cope Z. (1972) *The Acute Abdomen in Rhyme*. 5th edn. London, Lewis.

Deans G.T., McGalliard J.N. and Rutherford W.H. (1986) Incidence and duration of neck pain among patients injured in car accidents. *Br. Med. J.*, **292**, 94–5.

De Lacey G., Barker A., Wignall B. et al. (1979) Reasons for requesting radiographs in an accident department. *Br. Med. J.*, **1**, 1595–7.

Eastwood, H.D.H. (1987) Delayed diagnosis of femoral neck fracture in the elderly. *Age and Aging*, **16**, 378–82.

Editorial (1977) Reducing doctors' errors. *Br. Med. J.*, **1**, 1178.

Flatt A.E. (1979) *The Care of Minor Hand Injuries*. 4th edn, St. Louis, Mosby.

Galbraith S. (1976) Misdiagnosis and delayed diagnosis in traumatic intracranial haematoma. *Br. Med. J.*, **1**, 1438–39.

Guly H.R. (1986) Fractures not X-rayed. *Arch. Emerg. Med.*, **3**, 159–62.

Harvey I.M. and Roberts C.J. (1987) Clinical guidelines, medical litigation and the current medical defence system. *Lancet*, **i**, 145–47.

Holder A.R. (1972) Non negligent failure to take X-ray films. *JAMA*, **219**, 1259–60.

Illingworth C.M. (1975) Pulled elbow: a study of 100 patients. *Br. Med. J.*, **2**, 672–74.

Leaman A. (1986) 'Walking wounded' patients — how much history is necessary. *Br. J. Acc. Emerg. Med.*, March **1**, 12.

McCartney F.J. (1987) Diagnostic logic. *Br. Med. J.*, **295**, 1325–31.

Medical Defence Union Annual Report 1983. London Medical Defence Union, p. 19.

Melzack R., Wall P.D. and Ty T.C. (1982) Acute pain in an emergency clinic: latency of onset and descriptor patterns related to different injuries. *Pain*, **14**, 33–43.

Morgan W.J., Ogden E.C., Martin A. et al.(1980) Correlation between clinical and radiological diagnosis for fractures and dislocations in an accident department. *Injury* , **11**, 225–27.

Phillips G.D. and Baggoley C.H. (1986) The scientific basis of severe acute pain management in the emergency department. *Arch. Emerg. Med.*, **3**, 4–15.

Royal College of Radiologists Working Party (1985) Radiography of injured arms and legs in eight accident and emergency units in England and Wales. *Br. Med. J.*, **291**, 1325–28.

Warren R.A. and Fergusson D.G. (1984) Why do accident and emergency doctors request X-rays? *Arch. Emerg. Med.*, **1**, 143–50.

Wilson P.D., Jacobs B. and Schecter L. (1965) Slipped capital femoral epiphysis. *J. Bone Jt Surg.*, **47A**, 1128–45.

3　X-rays

INCIDENCE OF INJURIES MISSED ON X-RAY

The most common reason for missing injuries is by failing to diagnose fractures which are visible on X-rays (Guly, 1984). Many studies have looked at this (Table 3.1) and the number of missed diagnoses, expressed as a percentage of the total X-rays, has been found to vary between 0.8% (Galasco and Monahan, 1971) and 5.5% (Warren and Fergusson, 1984). Those figures hide much variation between X-rays of different areas of the body, and the most common areas in which injuries are missed when figures are expressed in this way are the extremities (elbow, wrist, hand, ankle and foot) (Wardrope and Chennells, 1985; Gleadhill, Thompson and Simms, 1987) and the face and skull (Wardrope and Chennells).

Table 3.1 Percentage of X-rays in which an abnormality was missed in an A & E department

Study	Percentage
Galasco and Monahan (1971)	0.8
Tachakra and Beckett (1985)	1.1
Swain (1986)	2.3
Welch and Renton (1979)	2.4
Vincent et al. (1988)	2.8
Carew-McColl (1983)	3.3
de Lacey et al. (1980)	3.5
Grech (1981)	3.8 includes false positives
Berman et al. (1985)	4.2
Mucci (1983)	4.4
Gleadhill, Thompson and Simms (1987)	4.9
Wardrope and Chennells (1985)	5
Warren and Fergusson (1984)	5.5

The importance of these missed injuries will depend on what the injury is, and only between a quarter and a half of these injuries are serious (de Lacey et al., 1980; Mucci, 1983; Gleadhill, Thompson and Simms, 1987). The incidence of significant missed injuries as a percentage of total X-rays has been found to be 2.3% (Mucci, 1983) and 2.5% (de Lacey et al., 1980) with the highest incidence of injuries of clinical importance being of the elbow, wrist and ankle (Gleadhill, Thompson and Simms, 1987), the face and skull (Wardrope and Chennells, 1985).

These small percentages, however, give a false picture because of the low incidence of many injuries. Vincent et al. (1988) found a missed diagnosis rate of 2.8%, which corresponds to the other studies, but these missed injuries actually made up 35% of all X-ray abnormalities and 39% of significant abnormalities. This rate varied between doctors. Another study showed 13% of positive findings were missed (Carew-McColl, 1983).

The more serious a potential injury is, the more likely the doctor is to X-ray the patient, and so the smaller the percentage of positive X-rays is likely to be. This, too, contributes to a false picture as, although only 0.5% of skull X-rays may be misinterpreted (Gleadhill, Thompson and Simms, 1987), in fact the percentage of fractures missed is between 9.2% (Gorman, 1987) and 60% (Vincent et al., 1988), (see also Chapter 6). When missed X-rays are calculated as a percentage of abnormalities, the highest incidence of missed injuries is in the skull, ankle, spine, hand and foot (Vincent et al., 1988).

WHY ARE INJURIES MISSED ON X-RAY?

Grech (1981) gives the reasons as:

1. Requesting the wrong X-ray
2. Defective radiographic techniques
3. Poor quality radiographs
4. Inexperience, misreading of overlapping anatomical shadows or artefacts and inadequate anatomical knowledge

The most common cause of all is insufficient care in examining the X-rays (Tachakra and Beckett, 1985), which I divide up as follows:

5. (a) Failure to look at every film
   (b) Failure to look at the whole film
   (c) Failure to look at the film as a whole
   (d) Forgetting to look at the soft tissues

6. Lastly, some X-ray changes are very subtle and difficult to detect (Tahakra and Beckett, 1985).

1. Requesting the wrong X-ray

This occurs either because the site of the injury has been wrongly localized or because of lack of thought when requesting X-rays. Abnormalities are shown best when they are in the centre of the X-ray field. Thus a wrist fracture will more easily be seen on a wrist X-ray then on an X-ray of the radius and ulna. The site of the injury should be localized and an X-ray taken of that area. If a patient has both wrist and elbow injuries, both joints need X-raying, rather than hoping to see both at either end of a forearm X-ray (but beware: it is not unknown to have X-rayed the elbow and upper forearm and the wrist and lower forearm and for there to have been a fracture in the middle inch of radius or ulna which was not X-rayed!).

It is also important that, where possible, one gets two X-rays at right angles, both to diagnose the injury and to assess any deformity. Thus a finger injury needs finger X-rays (i.e. an AP and a lateral of the finger) as hand X-rays (usually an AP or an oblique) may miss important fractures or dislocations of the proximal interphalangeal joint. Even if the patient has injured three fingers, each should be X-rayed individually rather than try to economise by doing one hand X-ray.

Some injuries (e.g. a fractured scaphoid) may need special views to demonstrate them. While doctors should try to learn which views are available (see later in the chapters devoted to different parts of the body), if the X-ray request form is filled in properly, stating what injury is suspected or what you wish to exclude, the radiographer should do the required views even without their being specifically requested.

2. Poor radiographic techniques

This usually relates to such factors as exposure problems, failing to ensure a true lateral of the elbow or ankle or doing facial X-rays AP rather than PA. Rarely the wrong side or the wrong digit may be X-rayed.

Radiographers will naturally be reluctant to inflict pain by moving an injured patient or an injured limb. If the patient is wheeled to X-ray lying down, a supine chest X-ray will be done rather than the much more informative erect X-ray. An uninterpretable lateral X-ray of the shoulder will be easier to do than abducting the arm to do an axial X-ray. The radiographer must ask whether a patient can be sat up or moved, and the doctor requesting an X-ray must be prepared to go into the X-ray room and (with the use of analgesia if necessary) put the patient into the position that the radiographer requires to do the X-rays. If it is not possible to get these X-rays, the doctor can discuss alternative views with the radiographer.

It is essential that X-rays are taken in at least two planes (at right angles if possible) even though, at times, this may be difficult in the injured patient, e.g. the axial shoulder X-ray mentioned above or a lateral X-ray of the hip. Failure to do this will ensure that injuries are missed. A lateral cervical spine X-ray by itself is not adequate for excluding a neck injury (Ross et al., 1987).

3. Poor quality X-rays

X-rays may be of poor quality because of poor radiographic technique or for other reasons, such as an unco-operative patient, severe pain or deformity, leading to difficulties is positioning, and obesity, leading to exposure problems. Portable X-ray machines usually provide X-rays of poorer quality than static equipment, which should always be used if possible.

In a series of head injured patients who were X-rayed, 27% had at least one unsatisfactory film (Swann, MacMillan and Strang, 1981) and a much higher percentage of cervical spine X-rays were of poor quality (Annis et al., 1987; Ross et al., 1987; Bryan, 1988), particularly in that they failed to demonstrate the cervicodorsal junction; this is a major cause of missed spine injuries (Braakman and Vinken, 1968; Ravichandran and Silver, 1982).

It is important that doctors are taught to recognize when an X-ray is of poor quality, so that they can discuss it with the radiographer. It may be that the films can be repeated or alternative views can be done but, depending on circumstances, it may be necessary to treat the patient without X-ray confirmation of the injury and then repeat the X-rays later when the patient is more cooperative or in a more stable condition.

4. Misreading of overlapping structures or artefacts

This is usually a cause of false positive diagnoses (see Chapter 1), while *inexperience* is a cause of both false positive and missed diagnoses, and is discussed in Chapter 5.

5. Insufficient care in examining X-rays

(a) On getting X-rays back, it is essential that every X-ray is taken from the packet. Nature being what it is, one can be sure that the one film left in the packet will be the only view that shows the fracture or at least it will be the view that demonstrates it best.

(b) It is essential that the whole X-ray film is looked at — not just the part where you suspect an injury. As discussed in Chapter 2, it is unfortunately common for the site of the injury to have been wrongly localized or the fracture site may not correspond to the area of maximum tenderness (Tachakra and Beckett, 1985) and it is very common for a fracture at the periphery of an X-ray to be missed (e.g. a scaphoid fracture visible at the periphery of an X-ray of the radius and ulna or a fractured fifth metatarsal base seen on an ankle X-ray).

Incidental findings on X-ray are common and, in one series, 1.6% of all X-rays had an incidental finding missed by the casualty officer but reported by the radiologist (Warren and Fergusson, 1984). These are usually of little importance (e.g. a small metallic foreign body in the hand of an engineering worker, degenerative change in a joint, calcification of an artery or a fibroid, an old fracture, etc.), but nothing can be dismissed as unimportant unless it is first seen, noted and diagnosed. Occasionally the incidental finding is much more important than the presenting injury, the most common significant incidental finding probably being a carcinoma or some other problem seen on a chest X-ray taken after a minor injury. If when looking at an X-ray one goes round the edge of every bone with a pencil or finger tip, it is really very difficult to miss fractures. Greenstick fractures are often missed and so, as well as looking for a line across a bone or the cortical break which signifies a fracture, it is also important to note the angulation or buckling of the cortex which occurs in this injury.

It is important that this process of going round the edge of every bone does not stop when a fracture has been found as there may be more than one fracture, and it is common in these circumstances for one or more fractures to be missed (Guly, 1984).

(c) It is also important to stand back and look at the X-ray film as a whole. Only then will a generalized abnormality such as an osteoporosis be noted. This will also prevent gross abnormalities being missed by devoting too much attention to the fine detail, as when a doctor examined a shoulder X-ray to exclude a fracture at such close range that he failed to spot an anterior dislocation (personal knowledge).

(d) Lastly the soft tissues must be looked at. Not only is a soft-tissue abnormality sometimes the only or the most obvious sign of an injury (e.g. prevertebral swelling in a cervical spine injury

(Gopalakrishnan and El Masri, 1986), the fat pad sign in elbow injuries (Smith and Lee, 1978), a liparthrosis in the knee or surgical emphysema of the orbit signifying a facial fracture, etc.) but in other injuries the soft tissue swelling will frequently indicate the position of a bony injury on the X-ray.

6. Subtle changes on X-ray

The X-ray appearances of some fractures may be subtle. Some of the classical difficult radiological diagnoses are listed in Table 3.2 and the specific injuries are discussed in relevant chapters later.

Even more subtle may be the X-ray appearances of some chest injuries (e.g. ruptured aorta or pneumothorax in the supine patient) and abdominal injuries (e.g. retroperitoneal air or intraperitoneal blood).

Table 3.2 Classical difficult radiological diagnoses

Cervical spine injury
Posterior dislocation of the shoulder (on AP view)
Dislocation of the lunate
Carpometacarpal dislocation
Scaphoid fracture
Slipped upper femoral epiphysis (on AP view)
Fractured calcaneum (on lateral X-ray of ankle)
Tarsometatarsal dislocation

If a patient has a dislocation reduced, it is of vital importance that another X-ray is done, partly to confirm that the reduction is complete but also because associated fractures may not be visible on the X-rays taken while the joint is dislocated, but will show on the post-reduction X-ray.

X-RAY REPORTING

I have already noted the incidence of missed diagnoses when X-rays are looked at by casualty officers and so it is essential that all A & E X-rays are reviewed by another person as, although he, too, may make mistakes, he will tend to miss different injuries.

Thus, in one series, casualty officers missed abnormalities in 4.2% of X-rays and radiographers in 4.5%, but both together missed abnormalities in only 2.3% (Berman et al., 1985).

This X-ray review will usually be done by a radiologist. These too may make errors (Table 3.3) but, like the errors of the casualty officer, these are not all significant. When X-rays are looked at by both casualty officers and radiologists only 0.2% (Galasco and Monahan, 1971) and 0.75% (de Lacey et al., 1980) of X-rays had injuries missed.

Table 3.3 Percentage of X-rays in which an abnormality was missed by a radiologist

Study	Percentage
Galasco and Monahan (1971)	0.4
Swain (1986)	1.9
de Lacey et al. (1980)	4
	(including false positives)
Rhea, Potsaid and De Luca (1979)	9.9
	(trainee radiologists)

The reasons why radiologists miss abnormalities have been looked at, and influencing factors include inexperience (Craig, 1981), with first-year radiology trainees making more errors than second-year trainees, poor quality films (again) and lack of clinical information (Rhea, Potsaid, and De Luca, 1979). Another study (Berbaum et al., 1988) has also shown that the diagnostic accuracy of radiologists is better if they are given clinical information than if they look at X-rays without this information. Inadequate viewing arrangements, fatigue and lack of interest have also been quoted as factors contributing to radiologists' errors, as have slips of memory due to hurried work (Craig, 1981). Finally, the radiologist may diagnose the injury himself but, because of unclear diction or other factors, there may be transcription errors leading to a wrong X-ray report.

When X-rays are reported, it is essential that a mechanism exists for comparing the radiologist's and the clinician's diagnosis as problems arise if the X-ray report is filed without being seen.

When an X-ray report of a missed fracture is received the patient's management will often not be altered, either because the fracture is minor and there is no specific treatment or the patient may have had the correct treatment anyway, and occasionally because, by the time the X-ray report is received, it is too late to alter treatment. For this reason it can be argued that those X-ray reports which seldom alter a patient's management (e.g. shoulder, fingers, toes, long bones) (Wardrope and Chennells, 1985) do not need to be reported. While this may be so in general terms, individual patients may suffer and a correct diagnosis is important for the reasons stated in Chapter 1. It is also important that doctors get feed-back on their clinical performance, as this will improve their diagnostic accuracy.

Practical points

● Give as much clinical detail as possible on your X-ray request form, including your clinical diagnosis. Not only will this assist the radiographer in choosing correct views, but it will also assist the radiologist who reports the X-ray.
● Be specific when you request X-rays so that the part you are interested in is in the centre of the X-ray.
● Do not accept poor quality X-rays without discussion with the radiographer as to how better films can be obtained.
● Go round the edge of every bone on the X-ray with a finger or a pencil, and do not stop when you find a fracture.
● Use an X-ray viewing screen and a bright light where necessary. Do not just hold X-rays up to the light or up to the window.
● Familiarize yourself with the appearances of the classically easily missed fractures.
● If in doubt, ask advice from someone more senior or a radiologist.
● If X-rays have been reported – always read the report, but look at the X-rays yourself as well.

REFERENCES

Annis J.A.D., Finlay D.B.L., Allen M.J. et al. (1987) A review of cervical spine radiographs in casualty patients. *Br. J. Radiol.,* **60,** 1059–61.

Berbaum K.S., El Khoury G.Y., Franken E.H. et al. (1988) Impact of clinical history on fracture detection with radiography. *Radiology,* **168,** 507–11.

Berman L., de Lacey G., Twomey E. et al. (1985) Reducing errors in the accident department: a simple method using radiographers. *Br. Med. J.,* **290,** 421–2.

Braakman R. and Vinken P.J. (1968) Old luxations of the lower cervical spine. *J. Bone Jt Surg.,* **50B,** 52–60.

Bryan A.S. (1988) A review of cervical spine X-rays from a casualty department. *J. R. Coll. Surg. Edinb.,* **33,** 143–5.

Carew-McColl M. (1983) Radiological interpretation in an accident and emergency department. *Br. J. Clin. Pract.,* **37,** 375–7.

Craig O. (1981) Emergency radiology. In *Problems in the Accident and Emergency Department.* London, Medical Protection Society, pp. 4–12.

de Lacey G., Barker A., Harper J. et al. (1980) An assessment of the clinical effects of reporting accident and emergency radiographs. *Br. J. Radiol.,* **53,** 304–9.

Galasco C.S.B. and Monahan P.R.W. (1971) Value of re-examining X-ray films of outpatients attending accident services. *Br. Med. J.,* **1,** 643–4.

Gleadhill D.N.S., Thompson J.Y. and Simms P. (1987) Can more efficient use be made of X-ray examinations in the accident and emergency department? *Br. Med. J.,* **294,** 943–7.

Gopalakrishnan K.C. and El Masri W. (1986) Prevertebral soft tissue shadow widening — an important sign of cervical spinal injury. *Injury,* **17,** 125–8.

Gorman D.F. (1987) The utility of post-traumatic skull X-rays. *Arch. Emerg. Med.,* **4,** 141–150.

Grech P. (1981) *Casualty Radiology. A Practical Guide for Radiological Diagnosis.* London, Chapman and Hall, p. 5.

Guly H.R. (1984) Missed diagnoses in an accident and emergency department. *Injury,* **15,** 403–6.

Mucci B. (1983) The selective reporting of X-ray films from the accident and emergency department. *Injury,* **14,** 343–4.

Ravichandran G. and Silver J.R. (1982) Missed injuries of the spinal cord. *Br. Med. J.,* **1,** 953–6.

Rhea J.T., Potsaid M.S. and De Luca S.A. (1979) Errors of interpretation as elicited by a quality audit of an emergency radiology facility. *Radiology,* **132,** 277–80.

Ross S.E., Schwab W., David E.T. et al. (1987) Clearing the cervical spine: initial radiologic evaluation. *J. Trauma,* **27,** 1055–60.

Smith D.N. and Lee J.R. (1978) The radiological diagnosis of post-traumatic effusion of the elbow joint and its clinical significance: the 'displaced fat pad' sign. *Injury,* **10,** 115–9.

Swain A.H. (1986) Radiological audit — changes in casualty officer performance during tenure of post. *Br. J. Acc. Emerg. Med.,* **1,** (June) 5–9.

Swann I.J., MacMillan R. and Strang I. (1981) Head injuries at an inner city accident and emergency department. *Injury,* **12,** 274–8.

Tachakra S.S. and Beckett M.W. (1985) Why do casualty officers miss radiological abnormalities? *J. R. Coll. Surg. Edinb.,* **30,** 311–3.

Vincent V.A., Driscoll P.A., Audley R.J. et al. (1988) Accuracy of detection of radiographic abnormalities by junior doctors. *Arch. Emerg. Med.,* **5,** 101–9.

Wardrope J. and Chennells P.M. (1985) Should all casualty radiographs be reviewed? *Br. Med. J.,* **240,** 1638–40.

Warren R.A. and Fergusson D.G. (1984) Why do accident and emergency doctors request X-rays? *Arch. Emerg. Med.,* **1,** 143–150.

Welch T.P. and Renton P. (1979) The value of radiological investigations in an accident and emergency department. *Br. J. Clin. Pract.,* **33,** 133–4.

4   Errors in the final diagnosis

THE FINAL DIAGNOSIS

The final diagnosis is made not just on the X-ray but on the history and examination as well. It is important to compare the X-ray diagnosis with the previously made provisional diagnosis and, while these will, hopefully, match, any great difference needs to be considered or the final diagnosis will be incorrect.

If the provisional diagnosis was of a minor injury but the patient seems to have a significant fracture or dislocation, this usually indicates that the clinical method was faulty, and so the patient should be re-examined in the light of this new evidence. There may, however, be alternative explanations. Firstly, the X-ray diagnosis may be incorrect and the 'fracture' may be an epiphysis, a nutrient artery or some other normal variant.

The next possibility is that the fracture is not recent. Most old fractures can be distinguished by callus formation or a periosteal reaction, and a longstanding non-union (e.g. of the scaphoid) will usually have rounded bone edges rather than the sharp ones of a recent fracture. Old skull fractures, however, may be indistinguishable from recent ones. The patient may be able to give details about previous injuries, or a search of old hospital notes or X-rays may prove that the injury is old. The finding of an unexplained old fracture in a child, together with a more recent injury, would suggest the possibility of non-accidental injury.

Longstanding dislocations may also present as new injuries (Guly, 1983) and there may be no radiological evidence to suggest the age of the injury. Errors are especially likely to occur if the patient is confused or unable to give an account of himself. Again, if there is any suspicion that the injury may be longstanding, previous hospital notes and X-rays should be looked for.

If the patient has had a significant fracture following minor trauma, it is possible that it is a pathological fracture in which case the final diagnosis must include a diagnosis of the cause of the bone weakness.

DIAGNOSING THE CAUSE OF THE INJURY

The final diagnosis must also include a diagnosis of the cause of the injury as this may be more important than the injury itself. An old person with a fractured neck of femur may have tripped, but there may be some other cause for the fall, such as postural hypotension or a cardiac arrhythmia, which may need investigation and treatment. If this is only considered days later, when the patient is having difficulty rehabilitating postoperatively, it will be impossible to determine why the fall occurred. It is therefore essential that this is investigated on admission. Many injuries are alcohol related and, unless this is diagnosed and the information communicated to the general practitioner, it is difficult for the patient to be helped.

The diagnosis of a patient with self-inflicted injuries must include, not just an accurate diagnosis of the wound and its complications, but also a diagnosis of why he cut himself and of any risk of suicide. The severity of the wound is not related to the severity of any psychiatric illness (Maloney, Shah and Fergusson, 1987).

Artefactual disease (e.g. swelling of the hand due to ligature application) will be missed if one is not suspicious (Smith, 1975).

NON-ACCIDENTAL INJURIES (NAI)

Other causes of injury which may not immediately be obvious, but where the cause may be more important than the injury itself, are non-accidental injuries resulting from wife battering, granny battering (elder abuse) (Council on Scientific Affairs, 1987) and child abuse.

It is vitally important that non-accidental injuries to children are not missed. In the A & E department it is very much a diagnosis made by comparing the objective findings of physical examination and X-ray with the history of how these injuries were meant to have been caused. It is important to be aware of what a child is capable of doing at any age and also of how injuries may be caused. Thus, a 2-month-old child is immobile and will not roll off a table while its nappy is being changed. Toddlers frequently fall, and spiral tibial fractures in this age group are common, but the same injury in a child who is not weight-bearing would be very suspicious of NAI.

Although most non-accidental injuries are identical to accidental injuries and it may be difficult to differentiate between them, there are some injuries which are very characteristic of NAI, e.g.

abrasions and small bruises of the face
torn frenulum of the lip and bruising of the gums
bruising of the pinna from pinching
finger tip bruising
subconjunctival and retinal haemorrhages
bite marks
cigarette burns
burns of the perineum or feet from 'dipping'
bruises or other injuries of different ages
patterned bruises, e.g. from a whip or a stick
rib fractures
radiological evidence of multiple injuries, especially of
    different ages
other evidence of neglect or failure to thrive.

Other factors raising suspicion include:
delay in seeking medical attention following an injury
multiple previous attendances at an A & E department
unusual parental behaviour or an unusual reaction to the
    child's injury

an inadequate history of the injury or else a history which
has clearly been rehearsed
previous history of abuse of the child or of a sibling.

Although all doctors are now aware of NAI, suspicion of it is
often based on prejudice. It may easily (too easily?) be considered in
the child of a harassed teenage single mother living in poor
conditions, but in the children of well-off, articulate parents it is still
very easy to fall into the trap described below:

'I was shown children with diagnoses... which simply were
examples of either ignorance or denial, I thought very much
the latter. I was shown children who had thrived for seven
months and then developed 'spontaneous subdural haematoma'... 'multiple bruises of unknown aetiology who had no
bleeding disorders and who did not bruise on the ward even
when they fell; 'osteogenesis imperfecta tarda' in kids who
had normal bones by X-ray, except that they showed on the
whole body X-ray many healing fractures which could be
dated; 'impetigo' in kids with skin lesions which were
clearly cigarette burns; 'accidental burns of buttocks in
symmetrical form, which could only occur from dunking a
child who had soiled into a bucket of hot water to punish
soiling... — these were all inflicted accidents or injuries.'
(Kempe, 1984).

Although the commonest reason for denial of the diagnosis is
the doctor's inability to believe that the parents (with whom the
doctor identifies) would be capable of inflicting the injuries, the
diagnosis may also be denied because of laziness or cowardice. To
dress a wound or to apply a plaster to a fracture may take 15
minutes, but the time and effort to investigate a case of non-
accidental injury and to follow it through to a case conference, and
possibly court, is considerable. Explaining to parents why you wish
to do further tests or to admit the child to hospital, or to confront
them with your suspicions, is not a pleasant task, but it is one which
must be faced for the benefit of the child.

It is equally important not to over-diagnose NAI as this may
cause great distress and family break-up (Paterson, 1986). This

usually occurs because of failure to elicit the history properly and by starting off by being hostile to the parents (Kirschner and Stein, 1985). Some conditions which may be mistaken for child abuse are listed in Table 4.1, and those conditions which may be mistaken for burns are described in Chapter 21.

Table 4.1 Some conditions which may mimic child abuse (Kirschner and Stein, 1985; Wheeler and Hobbs, 1988) (this is not a complete list)

Bleeding disorders
    Haemophilia
    Idiopathic thrombocytopenic purpura
    Haemolytic disease of the newborn

Conditions simulating bruising
    Mongolian blue spot
    Post mortem lividity
    Subconjunctival haemorrhage due to pertussis
    Facial swelling of other causes, e.g. post dental
        treatment and allergic periorbital swelling
    Folk medicine, e.g. cupping

Other causes of fractures
    Osteogenesis imperfecta
    Copper deficiency
    Birth injury

Conditions simulating recent fracture
    Congenital variation of skull sutures
    Caffey's disease
    Osteomyelitis

Others
    Alopecia areata

A significant percentage of children with osteogenesis imperfecta are initially misdiagnosed as being victims of NAI (Paterson and McAllion, 1987), though some doubt has been cast on the criteria used to establish the diagnosis in this series (Carty and Shaw, 1988; Taitz, 1987). Features of osteogenesis imperfecta include blue sclerae, a family history and progressive deformity. As long as the possibility is considered, the diagnosis should not be missed (but frequently is). The major difficulty is with children who have a sporadic type IV osteogenesis imperfecta without any of these features, but this is very rare, with a large city having one case every 100–300 years (Taitz, 1987).

Copper deficiency too is a rare condition which may (but should not) be confused with NAI (Chapman, 1987; Shaw, 1988). Copper deficiency, being a metabolic bone disease, affects the whole skeleton and is symmetrical. Skull fractures do not occur and, in addition, there are other features such as anaemia, pallor and hypotonia.

Most genital injuries in girls present with a clear history of trauma, especially of a 'falling astride' injury, but sexual abuse needs to be considered in the occasional patient. However, most cases of sexual abuse do not present as acute injuries. Lichen sclerosis et atrophicus may masquerade as sexual abuse (Handfield-Jones, Hinde and Kennedy, 1987), but its diagnosis does not exclude the possibility of abuse (Davidson, Clarke and Kean, 1987).

Practical points

● Whenever you see an injured child, always ask yourself whether the injury is compatible with the history given. If not, consider NAI.

● If you suspect NAI, search for records of previous attendances at A & E, examine the child from head to toe, check the NAI register and seek advise as your local guidelines suggest.

NON-TRAUMATIC CONDITIONS PRESENTING FOLLOWING INJURY

A history of injury will usually lead to a diagnosis of some traumatic condition, but it is important to consider other diseases, as many patients with non-traumatic conditions will also give a history of injury.

This occurs in three circumstances:

1. The injury draws attention to a pre-existing condition
2. The injury has an aetiological role in a condition usually considered non-traumatic
3. Coincidence

If a condition causes few symptoms or is very slowly progressive, the patient may not realize that it exists until an injury draws attention to it, and he may genuinely believe it to have been caused by the injury. (Beware, however, of the rare, but mischievous, patient who deliberately hides his past history and tries to claim compensation for it following an accident.) The true diagnosis is usually obvious but occasionally doctors, too, may make mistakes. Thus breast carcinoma may be misdiagnosed as traumatic fat necrosis, tumours may be mistaken for haematomas (Cross, 1985; Guly, 1986) and tendon or joint injuries may be considered as a cause for a hand deformity before a correct diagnosis of Dupuytren's contracture is made. Conditions mimicking non-accidental injuries have been described earlier.

The symptoms of a chronic condition, such as ankylosing spondylitis, may date from an injury (Jacoby, Newell and Hickling, 1985). An X-ray taken at that time may show that X-ray abnormalities already existed but, on occasion, there may have been no manifestation of the disease prior to the injury. It is usually considered that the injury has merely unmasked the ankylosing spondylitis, possibly because the rest prescribed for the injury has worsened the spondylitis (Jacoby, Newell and Hickling). However, it has been postulated that the trauma may have a role in the aetiology of the spondylitis in this very small number of patients (Masson et al., 1985).

Trauma is an aetiological factor in infective conditions. Thus septic bursitis may follow a blunt injury, and a history of trauma is common in children with osteomyelitis. Tuberculous bone and joint infections may also follow trauma (Ferris, Goldie and Weir, 1987) and these conditions may be diagnosed late if only traumatic causes are considered for the symptoms.

Reiter's disease too may rarely present following an injury and a possible causative role has been postulated (Wisnieski, 1984; Masson et al., 1985).

Minor injuries are very common, especially in children, and so an association between onset of symptoms and an injury may be entirely coincidental. If a child develops a headache and drowsiness 24 hours after a head injury (however minor), the symptoms are likely to be blamed on the injury, and so there may be a delay in diagnosing the meningitis or other condition that the child is really suffering from.

Practical points

● Just because the patient had an injury and now has symptoms, this does not mean that the two are necessarily related. Keep an open mind and consider other possibilities.

IF A BONY INJURY IS SUSPECTED CLINICALLY BUT THE X-RAY IS NORMAL

The fact that the X-rays appear normal does not exclude a serious injury. The names and the dates on the X-ray should be checked, as occasionally X-rays get muddled up or there may have been previous films in the packet. Check that the correct bit has been X-rayed, as it is not unknown for an X-ray of the wrong limb or digit to have been requested or done. The patient should also be re-examined to ensure that the site of injury has been correctly identified. If the doctor is still convinced that the patient should have a fracture but he cannot see it, advice should be sought and somebody more senior should review the X-rays.

Some injuries (e.g. a fractured calcaneum) may be difficult or even impossible to see on standard X-rays, and special views may be required. On occasions oblique X-rays may show a fracture at the ankle or the wrist much better than standard views.

Ligamentous injuries may be serious but will not show on standard X-rays. Some may be diagnosable clinically (e.g. in the hand or knee) but others may need stress X-rays (e.g. in the ankle).

Tendon injuries, too (e.g. patellar tendon rupture) will not show on X-ray.

Lastly, some other fractures may not show on initial X-rays and may not be visible until further X-rays at 10–14 days show either a more obvious fracture line due to bone resorption or else a periosteal reaction or callus. This may occur with many injuries but the more common ones are listed in Table 4.2 and are discussed elsewhere in their relevant chapters. If there is good clinical evidence of a fracture, many patients will need to be treated as if they have one until it can be proved that they do not. If it is important that an early diagnosis is made, a bone scan may be useful.

Table 4.2 Fractures which may not be visible on initial X-rays (see relevant chapters for details)

Scaphoid
Neck of femur
Radial head
Rib
Skull
Spiral fracture of tibia in toddlers
Stress fractures
Epiphyseal fractures

REFERENCES

Carty H. and Shaw D.G. (1988) Child abuse and osteogenesis imperfecta. *Br. Med. J.*, **296**, 292.

Chapman S. (1987) Child abuse or copper deficiency? A radiological view. *Br. Med. J.*, **294**, 1370.

Council on Scientific Affairs (1987) Elder abuse and neglect. *JAMA*, **257**, 966–71.

Cross A.B. (1985) Bronchogenic carcinoma presenting as an injured thumb. *Arch. Emerg. Med.*, **2**, 93–6.

Davidson D.C., Clarke M.D.B. and Kean H.B. (1987) Lichen sclerosis et atrophicus in children misdiagnosed as sexual abuse. *Br. Med. J.*, **295**, 211.

Ferris B.D., Goldie B. and Weir W. (1987) An unusual presentation of tuberculosis – 'Injury TB'. *Injury*, **18**, 347–9.

Guly H.R. (1983) Longstanding dislocations presenting as acute injuries. *Br. J. Acc. Emerg. Med.*, **1** (July), 13–14.

Guly H.R. (1986) Beware the 'haematoma'. *Br. J. Acc. Emerg. Med.*, **1** (June), 16.

Handfield-Jones S.E., Hinde F.R.J. and Kennedy C.T.C. (1987) Lichen sclerosis et atrophicus in children misdiagnosed as sexual abuse. *Br. Med. J.*, **294**, 1404–5.

Jacoby R.K., Newell R.L.M. and Hickling P. (1985) Ankylosing spondylitis and trauma: the medico-legal implications. A comparative study of patients with non-specific back pain. *Ann. Rheum. Dis.*, **44**, 307–11.

Kempe C.H. (1984) quoted by Heinz M. The battered child revisited. *JAMA*, **251**, 3295–300.

Kirschner R.H. and Stein R.J. (1985) The mistaken diagnosis of child abuse. *Am. J. Dis. Child.*, **139**, 873–5.

Maloney C., Shah S. and Fergusson D.G. (1987) Acute management of the self cutter. *Arch. Emerg. Med.*, **4**, 39–45.

Masson G., Thomas P., Bortoux D. et al. (1985) Influence of trauma on initiation of Reiter's syndrome and ankylosing spondylitis. *Ann. Rheum. Dis.*, **44**, 860–2.

Paterson C.R. (1986) Fractures in osteogenesis imperfecta. *Br. Med. J.*, **293**, 699.

Paterson C.R. and McAllion S.J. (1987) Child abuse and osteogenesis imperfecta. *Br. Med. J.*, **295**, 1561.

Shaw J.C.L. (1988) Copper deficiency and non-accidental injury. *Arch. Dis. Child.*, **63**, 448–55.

Smith R.J. (1975) Factious lymphedema of the hand. *J. Bone Jt Surg.*, **57A**, 89–94.

Taitz L.S. (1987) Child abuse and osteogenesis imperfecta *Br. Med. J.*, **295**, 1082–3.

Taitz L.S. (1988) Child abuse and osteogenesis imperfecta. *Br. Med. J.*, **296**, 292.

Wheeler D. and Hobbs C.J. (1988) Mistakes in diagnosing non-accidental injury: 10 years' experience. *Br. Med. J.*, **296**, 1233–6.

Wisnieski J.J. (1984) Trauma and Reiter's syndrome: development of 'reactive arthropathy' in two patients following musculoskeletal injury. *Ann. Rheum. Dis.*, **43**, 829–33.

5   Other factors

INJURIES IN CHILDREN

Injuries in small children may cause particular problems in their diagnosis.

Firstly, they will be unable to give a proper history themselves, which may result in the diagnostic problems previously mentioned. Toddlers are prone to falling down, but these falls may not all be witnessed. They may therefore have fractures to explain symptoms even in the absence of any history of injury. In one series of 500 children under 5 years with a limp of unknown aetiology, whose pelvis and whole lower limb were X-rayed, 100 (20%) were found to have fractures (Oudjhane et al., 1988). The problems of non-accidental injury have already been discussed (Chapter 4).

Physical examination of the child may be difficult as it may be impossible to localize tenderness (especially if the child is screaming) and the child will not cooperate in testing tendon and nerve function.

There is sometimes a reluctance to expose children to X-radiation, particularly to the pelvis. A lead shield to protect the gonads may hide fractures on the X-ray and so, while it may be used on follow-up X-rays, it should never be used on the initial diagnostic X-ray.

Children's X-rays may be difficult to interpret because of the variable appearance of the epiphyses at different ages. Clearly separation of unossified epiphyses cannot be diagnosed radiologically and in other epiphyses with a large amount of cartilage, the severity of the fracture may be greatly underestimated by the radiological displacement (e.g. fractures of the lateral condyle of the elbow). Many epiphyseal injuries are best diagnosed by observing that the epiphysis is not 'sitting' symmetrically on the metaphysis, and X-rays of the other side for comparison are often helpful. Some epiphyseal fractures (e.g. the lower femur, the upper tibia — see Chapter 16 — and the lower fibula) may have normal initial X-rays and need stress X-rays under general anaesthesia for their diagnosis (Rang, 1974).

Spiral fractures of the tibia (Chapter 16) may not be visible on initial X-rays, and minor greenstick fractures of long bones are frequently missed because the angulation or buckling of the cortex is not recognized for what it is.

Practical points

- A child who is not using its arm needs the whole upper limb examined, from the sternoclavicular joint to the finger tip, and a child not weight-bearing on a leg needs the lower limb examined from pelvis to toes.
- Physical examination of a happy child is much easier and more informative than that of a screaming child. Time spent putting the child at ease is well spent. If any of the examination is likely to be painful — save it to last. Concentrate initially on the parts you do not expect to find injured. Examine for tenderness early, as you cannot localize tenderness in a crying child, whereas you can test for range of joint movement in any child.
- If you are uncertain about X-ray appearances — X-ray the other side for comparison, and ask advice.
- If a child appears to have a significant knee injury but X-rays are normal — ask advice.
- If a child has a wound which, by its position, may have divided tendon or nerve and you cannot test these — the wound should be explored and repaired under general anaesthesia.

ALCOHOL

The consumption of alcohol contributes to many accidents and, if the patient is intoxicated, this may make the diagnosis of injuries very difficult. Alcohol has been reported as contributing to the misdiagnosis of many injuries, including severe head injuries (Jennett and Miller, 1972; Galbraith, 1976), spinal injuries (Hardy, 1977; Ravichandran and Silver, 1982; Reid et al., 1987), splenic injury (McLauchlan et al., 1988) and multiple injuries (Dearden and Rutherford, 1985).

The first problem is the effect of alcohol on the patient. At worst, the patient may be unable to give any history at all and so a traumatic cause of the problem may be overlooked. Even if less intoxicated, he may have poor recall, confused thinking and slurred speech. Alcohol, by its analgesic effect, may mask pain and tenderness, and the intoxicated patient is likely to be uncooperative both with physical and radiographic examination (Rix, 1987).

The patient's drunkenness may also have effects on the doctor, who may show an unfortunate (though possibly understandable) antagonism to a badly behaved drunk who is disrupting the A & E department and whose injuries are the result of his drunkenness. Antagonism towards a patient before one even starts to examine him is a sure way of overlooking important pathology.

Alcohol is a central nervous system depressant, but to attribute a diminished level of consciousness to alcohol may have fatal results. The diagnosis of many intracranial haematomas is missed or delayed because of this (Galbraith, 1976) (Chapter 6). In alcoholics, traumatic brain injuries severe enough to cause significant intellectual impairment may go unrecognized (Hillbom and Holm, 1986).

The clinical diagnosis of alcohol ingestion by detecting the smell of alcohol on the breath and by observing its effects on the patient's speech, eyes and coordination is inaccurate, with false positives and many false negatives (Rutherford, 1977). The only accurate way of diagnosing alcohol ingestion is to measure blood, breath or urinary alcohol levels. It has been shown that a blood alcohol level of less than 200 mg per 100 ml does not depress the level of consciousness, and a blood alcohol level of less than 300 mg per 100 ml should not cause coma (Rutherford, 1977). The converse is not true, and one should never attribute a depressed level of consciousness to alcohol in a head-injured patient. The effects of alcohol are very variable, and some patients with a very high blood alcohol level may be fully conscious (Redmond, 1986). Also the fact of a very high blood alcohol level does not exclude the possibility of an intracranial haematoma being present as well.

Similarly, alcohol intoxication may cause hypotension but, in the injured patient, one must always look for blood loss as a cause of the hypotension and never blame the alcohol alone (except in retrospect).

Practical points

- Do not diagnose drunkenness just by the smell of alcohol on the breath. A patient who has had one drink may smell as much as someone who has had ten.
- Do not forget the association between alcohol ingestion and hypoglycaemia.
- Every patient is entitled to your best care. Do not let your professionalism and standards slip for drunks, despite provocation.
- A diminished level of consciousness in the drunk head injury must *never* be attributed to the alcohol. Always assume that it is due to the head injury (except in retrospect).
- Hypotension must be assumed to be due to blood loss and not alcohol (except in retrospect).

RARITIES

Many of the diagnostic errors described in this book are rare injuries. In an A & E department of a size to employ six senior house officers changing every six months, it would be a rare day when a patient with a Colles fracture was not seen and a rare week that went by without seeing a patient with an anterior dislocation of the shoulder. All doctors should become proficient at diagnosing these injuries. However, this department may see only two posteriorly dislocated shoulders a year or one dislocated lunate. Other injuries are even rarer, being poorly described in basic textbooks and only mentioned in specialist texts not read by junior staff at this level. Therefore the majority of doctors working in the department will never see these injuries, but will still be expected to diagnose them if they occur. This problem of sustaining an observer's attention, so that an occasional abnormality is detected among a mass of normal results, has been addressed in other medical specialties such as cytology (Fowkes, 1986), where it has been confirmed that diagnostic sensitivity is less with a lower prevalence. Apart from obvious factors, such as experience, vigilance is also altered by the doctor's personality and by environmental factors, such as temperature and background noise. Vigilance also diminishes with increasing time on a shift.

LONGSTANDING NEUROLOGICAL DISEASE

Injuries may be very difficult to diagnose in patients with loss of sensation as a result of longstanding spinal cord injuries and diseases or other neurological injuries or problems (e.g. peripheral neuropathy) (Johnson, 1967). Not only is there loss of the sensation which usually draws attention to an injury, but loss of muscle power will lead to lack of any classical deformity due to the injury. Severe osteoporosis due to disuse will lead to pathological fractures with minimal or no trauma. Thus a fractured femur may be misdiagnosed as a deep vein thrombosis (Cocksedge, Freestone and Martin, 1984).

BAD LUCK

When investigating diagnostic errors, one frequently finds not one cause for the missed diagnosis but that minor problems have occurred at every stage of the diagnostic process, each one pointing the doctor a little further from the true diagnosis. Sometimes the probability of so many problems occurring in one particular patient is so small that, when the doctor finally misses the diagnosis, one cannot blame any individual, but can only conclude that it was the result of bad luck. Thus a patient with a communication problem, who has an uncommon presentation of a rare injury, and who attends the A & E department on a busy day, is X-rayed by an inexperienced radiographer, who doesn't get the projection quite right, and the X-rays are then interpreted by a very junior doctor, is almost certainly not going to be correctly diagnosed.

While bad luck is a factor in missed diagnoses, it should not be invoked as a cause too often!

ORGANIZATIONAL PROBLEMS

While significant misdiagnoses in A & E departments are usually blamed on individual doctor's failures in history taking, clinical examination, judgement or X-ray interpretation, the system which employs these doctors must take some of the blame for employing inexperienced doctors in this most difficult area and for failing to provide proper training, support and optimum working conditions.

Medical schools do not aim to produce competent clinicians but doctors 'with the knowledge, skills, attitudes and an understanding of principles to provide a basis for postgraduate training' (Walton, 1985). Many medical students have no specific attachment to A & E departments, and in those medical schools which do provide training in A & E it is usually fairly short. Radiology and orthopaedics, including teaching the examination of the musculoskeletal system, are not usually given great prominence in an overcrowded medical school curriculum. After qualifying, doctors spend a year obtaining experience of (usually) general medicine and general surgery before being thrown into the deep end of an A & E department, seeing, examining and interpreting the X-rays of patients of all ages and types, but mostly with injuries. It is hardly surprising that errors do occur.

INEXPERIENCE AND TRAINING

Inexperience is clearly a major factor in missed diagnoses, and this should be able to be rectified by formal training and 'on the job' experience, backed up by feedback on the errors made, but the extent to which this happens in practice is doubtful. Four studies have looked at casualty officers' abilities to interpret X-rays at different stages of their six-month appointment. Two studies have demonstrated that, as expected, the error rate is highest in the first month of appointment (Tachakra and Beckett, 1985; Vincent et al., 1988). Thereafter two studies show that the error rate is not improved during the rest of the appointment (Swain, 1986; Vincent et al., 1988), though one of these (Swain, 1986) notes a lessening of false positive diagnoses. One study (Gleadhill, Thompson and Simms, 1987) shows a steady improvement during the appointment, which the authors attribute to training and guidelines rather than to experience. A final study shows that the error rate is higher in the last month of a six-month appointment than in the second to fifth months (Tachakra and Beckett, 1985), demonstrating that, while inexperience may be important, it is clearly not the only or major factor.

It is therefore clear that just working in an A & E department does not in itself give the experience required to avoid diagnostic errors, but that this must be backed up by formal training. Most A & E departments do organize teaching programmes for their staff, though the value of these in improving diagnostic accuracy has not been tested. However, the knowledge and clinical skills required to work safely in an A & E department is extensive and really needs to be taught before doctors are allowed to work. Almost invariably this is not possible, and teaching needs to be done in the early weeks of an appointment, although this may be made difficult by staff starting on different dates and the problems of providing cover while teaching is being done. Teaching for one session per week throughout the six month appointment is common, but this does not help the patient with a dislocated lunate seen on a doctor's first day working in A & E!

STAFFING

The amount of backup and support for inexperienced doctors is increasing but is still variable. Some larger A & E departments may have several senior and middle-grade staff to give advice and a few may have an experienced doctor in the A & E department 24 hours a day, but many departments have just one or even no senior doctor. In these departments, the more seriously ill and injured can easily be referred to the duty specialist team, but there may be no one to turn to for advice on the seemingly minor musculoskeletal injury.

Not only are the numbers of more senior staff variable, but so are the numbers of junior doctors who, in most departments, see the majority of new patients. There is great variation in work patterns between A & E departments (e.g. in some all the suturing is done by doctors, in others, by nurses; medical problems take longer to deal with than minor trauma, etc.), making comparisons between departments difficult, but there is a two or threefold variation in 'patients seen per doctor hour' between hospitals (unpublished data from West Midlands 1983). These arrangements, by which doctors in one hospital are seeing double the numbers of patients in a given time than in another hospital, seem to be unplanned and to result from historical accident. Its relevance to errors in the department cannot be proved but can be guessed at, particularly as a study from general practice has demonstrated that patients given shorter appointments with a doctor had fewer problems identified and were less satisfied than patients with longer appointments (Morrell et al., 1986).

A & E departments should be adequately staffed with both doctors and other staff, to ensure that doctors are not put under pressure to take short cuts.

WORKING UNDER PRESSURE

Work in an A & E department cannot be planned and there is a great variation in work-load from day to day, which cannot always be matched to staffing levels. When an A & E department is very busy and patients are agitating in the waiting room, there is very great pressure on doctors to see patients quickly. While most people can work faster if they need to, inexperienced staff may find themselves taking short cuts in history and examination, and this almost invariably leads to errors. Also, when a department is busy, a doctor is more likely to be interrupted while seeing a patient in order to see a more seriously ill patient or to answer the telephone. He thus ends up treating two or three patients simultaneously, and this must lead to more errors or poor patient care in other ways. It must be admitted, however, that only a minority of errors occur when a doctor is stressed in this way (Tachakra and Beckett, 1985).

HAND-OVER

In any system where doctors work shifts to provide a 24-hour service, there must be occasions when one doctor sees a patient and then goes off duty, leaving another doctor to interpret the X-rays. It has been noted above that diagnosis is the product of both clinical and radiological findings, and so a formal hand-over must be made, notes must be perfect and the doctor interpreting the X-ray must re-examine the patient (Tachakra and Beckett, 1985).

FATIGUE

It is difficult to prove that tiredness in a doctor at the end of a long shift or following a heavy period of duty is a cause of diagnostic error, but it almost certainly is. Sleep disruption initially impairs short-term recall and will cause fatigue and mood changes (Deary and Tait, 1987; Durnford, 1988). This will influence efficiency in a team and inter-personal relationships, which must hinder communication that is so important in reaching a diagnosis. More prolonged sleep loss directly influences performance, and will cause doctors to forget to do routine and monotonous tasks. This must have an influence on all a doctor's functions, including his diagnostic ability.

PERSONALITY AND MOTIVATION

There is much individual variation in diagnostic ability between casualty officers (Swain, 1986; Gleadhill, Thompson and Simms, 1987; Vincent et al., 1988) and, while this may reflect intelligence and experience, there can be no doubt that personality, attitudes and motivation (Durnford, 1988) are very important, not just for this, but for all aspects of a doctor's work.

'In medicine the tragedies occur because doctors don't think, don't communicate clearly, can't be bothered or are ill...' (Mitchell, 1984)

Doctors' illness must be a rare cause of diagnostic error in the A & E department, but it must be acknowledged that doctors sometimes cannot be bothered, and this shows itself in A & E by regarding patients not as individuals but as a queue to be shifted, which invariably leads to short cuts and errors. A doctor's personality is all-important in the development of his overall attitude, but there will also be day-to-day variations, dependent on his personal and home life and working environment. Although it is difficult to prove, it stands to reason that the doctor who is happy and contented at work will do his job more efficiently and effectively (Rankin, Serieys and Elliott-Binns, 1987). The health authority must employ adequate staff in a safe and pleasant working environment, and senior A & E doctors must regard motivation of their staff as a very important part of their job.

REFERENCES

Cocksedge S., Freestone S. and Martin J.F. (1984) Unrecognised femoral fractures in patients with paraplegia due to multiple sclerosis. *Br. Med. J.*, **289**, 309.

Dearden C.H. and Rutherford W.H. (1985) The resuscitation of the severely injured in the accident and emergency department — a medical audit. *Injury*, **16**, 249–52.

Deary I.J. and Tait R. (1987) Effect of sleep disruption on cognitive performance and mood in medical house officers. *Br. Med. J.*, **295**, 1513–16.

Durnford S. (1988) Junior hospital doctors: tired and tested. *Br. Med. J.*, **297**, 931–2.

Fowkes F.G.R. (1986) Diagnostic vigilance. *Lancet*, **i**, 493–4.

OTHER FACTORS

OTHER FACTORS

Galbraith S. (1976) Misdiagnosis and delayed diagnosis in traumatic intracranial haematoma. *Br. Med. J.*, **1**, 1438–9.

Gleadhill D.N.S., Thompson J.Y. and Simms P. (1987) Can more efficient use be made of X-ray examinations in the accident and emergency department? *Br. Med. J.*, **294**, 943–7.

Hardy A.G. (1977) Cervical spinal cord injury without bony injury. *Paraplegia*, **14**, 296–305.

Hillbom M. and Holm L. (1986) Contribution of traumatic head injury to neuropsychological deficits in alcoholics. *J. Neurol. Neurosurg. Psychiatry*, **49**, 1348–53.

Jennett B. and Miller J.D. (1972) Infection after depressed fracture of the skull. *J. Neurosurg.*, **36**, 333–9.

Johnson J.T.H. (1967) Neuropathic fractures and joint injuries. *J. Bone Jt Surg.*, **49A**, 1–30.

McLauchlan C.A.J., Maheson M., Sloan J.P. et al. (1988) Towards earlier diagnosis of splenic injury. *Arch. Emerg. Med.*, **5**, 34–7.

Mitchell J.R.A. (1984) Who needs clinical pharmacology? *Br. Med. J.*, **289**, 1119–20.

Morrell D.C., Evans M.E., Morris R.W. et al. (1986) The 'five minute' consultation: effect of time constraint on clinical content and patient satisfaction. *Br. Med. J.*, **292**, 870–3.

Oudjhane K., Newman B., Oh K.S. et al. (1988) Occult fractures in pre-school children. *J. Trauma*, **28**, 858–60.

Rang M. (1974) *Children's Fractures*, 2nd edn, Philadelphia, Lippincott.

Rankin H.J., Serieys N.M. and Elliott-Binns C.P. (1987) Determinants of mood in general practitioners. *Br. Med. J.,*. **294**, 618–20.

Ravichandran G. and Silver J.R. (1982) Missed injuries of the spinal cord. *Br. Med. J.*, **284**, 953–6.

Redmond A.D. (1986) Central nervous system depression and high blood ethanol levels. *Lancet*, **i**, 805.

Reid D.C., Henderson R., Saboe L. et al. (1987) Etiology and clinical course of missed spine fractures. *J. Trauma*, **27**, 980–6.

Rix K.J.B. (1987) Problems associated with alcohol intoxication. *Hospital Update*, **13**, 1010–18.

Rutherford W.H. (1977) Diagnosis of alcohol ingestion in mild head injuries. *Lancet*, **i**, 1021–3.

Swain A.H. (1986) Radiological audit — change in casualty officer performance during tenure of post. *Br. J. Acc. Emerg. Med.*, June, 5–9.

Tachakra S.S. and Beckett M.W. (1985) Why do casualty officers miss radiological abnormalities? *J. R. Coll. Surg. Edinb.*, **30**, 311–13.

Vincent C.A., Driscoll P., Audley R.J. and Grant D.S. (1988) Accuracy of detection of radiographic abnormalities by junior doctors. *Arch. Emerg. Med.*, **5**, 101–9.

Walton J. (1985) Educating the doctor: basic education. *Br. Med. J.*, **290**, 1719–22.

6 Head injuries

IMPORTANCE OF DIAGNOSING SKULL FRACTURES

Discussion about the difficulties of diagnosing skull fractures must be prefaced by some comment as to whether this is important or not. In cases of closed head injury, the important factor is whether or not there is a brain injury or an intracranial haematoma, and these cannot be seen on a skull X-ray. A linear skull fracture may be complicated by an extradural haematoma but, in itself, causes no harm, merely showing that a significant force has been applied to the skull (though not necessarily to the brain).

Radiologists point out that, in patients having skull X-rays taken after trauma, the yield of fractures is low, the complication rate is very low and detecting a fracture does not alter management and so is of little value (Evans, 1977). The Royal College of Radiologists (1981) found, in a study of 4829 patients with uncomplicated head injuries, that only one developed an unexpected intracranial haematoma.

On the other hand, it has been demonstrated that the head injured patient with a skull fracture is 200 times more likely to suffer an intracranial haematoma than the patient without a fracture (Mendelow et al., 1983) and so neurosurgeons believe that their detection is crucial. Jennett (1987), in a brief review, argues that the importance of skull fractures is in the prediction of complications and not their diagnosis. Knowing that a patient does not have a skull fracture is also of value, as it allows the patient to be sent home in the knowledge that the risk of a complication is very small.

For the purposes of this chapter, I therefore accept that in patients with minor head injuries it is important that all skull fractures are detected to pick out those patients who need to be admitted and observed.

If a patient's condition is such that he needs admission anyway, finding a skull fracture will not alter immediate management and so, while an X-ray may still be done, it is not a priority. Attempts to get skull X-rays of diagnostic quality on a struggling and unco-operative patient are not worthwhile, and certainly investigation and treatment of other injuries (including investigation of brain injury with a CT scan) will always take precedence over trying to prove or disprove the presence of a skull fracture.

The majority of extradural haematomas will present within 24 hours, and so a patient with a minor head injury and skull fracture will usually stay in hospital for between two and seven days, depending on the clinician. Therefore a patient presenting three days following a head injury and found to have a skull fracture would, had the injury been diagnosed soon after it occurred, probably have been discharged from hospital already, and so detecting this fracture is of little clinical importance.

Practical points

● Skull X-rays do not need to be done on patients with old injuries (unless you suspect a compound depressed fracture).

SKULL FRACTURES

It is important to realize that some skull fractures may not be visible on standard skull X-rays. This has been demonstrated in a study on cadaver heads (Webber and Folio, 1976) and clinically. A study has been reported of 390 head injured patients who had scalp wounds explored with a gloved finger and sometimes a retractor, and also had skull X-rays. Thirteen skull fractures were detected in all, but only 4 were seen on skull X-rays. Wound exploration detected 11 (Fullarton et al., 1987). The occasional skull fracture not visible on standard X-rays (AP, Towne's and clinically indicated lateral) may be visible if both lateral X-rays are done (Leaman et al., 1988).

The significance of these fractures which cannot be seen on X-ray is uncertain. Some may be through one table of the skull only. Fractures through both tables may be less displaced than those readily seen on X-ray and may be associated with fewer complications, but this is unproven, and all skull fractures, however diagnosed, should be treated with equal importance as they may be associated with extradural haematomas.

In particular, fractures of the temporal bone which may be associated with injuries to the seventh and eighth cranial nerves and CSF otorrhoea may not be visible on standard skull X-rays, and so may be missed (Waldron and Hurley, 1988). However, they should be detected on examination of the ears (e.g. blood in the external auditory meatus or behind the tympanic membrane or a 'step' in the wall of the external auditory maetus) and on tuning fork tests. Even if a fracture in another part of the skull vault is seen on X-ray, these tests should still be done as temporal fractures not visible on X-ray may be associated with other fractures.

Other fractures of the base of the skull which, being open fractures, carry the risk of intracranial infection as a complication may also not be visible on standard skull X-rays and should be diagnosed on clinical grounds (Table 6.1), and the lateral skull X-ray should be looked at for evidence of a fluid level in the ethmoid sinus.

Table 6.1 Signs of a fractured base of skull

CSF rhinorrhoea or otorrhoea

Bleeding from the ear or haemotympanum

Bilateral black eyes in the absence of local injury

Bruising over the mastoids

Fluid level in the ethmoid sinus on lateral skull X-ray

Le Fort II and III middle third facial fractures are often associated with basal skull fractures and CSF rhinorrhoea.

Practical points

● All scalp wounds should, if long enough, be explored with a gloved finger and the skull inspected, using a retractor if necessary, and any fractures detected in this way should be treated in the same way as fractures detected on X-rays.
● Examination of the ears with an auriscope and tuning fork tests should be part of the routine examination of all head injured patients.

WHO REQUIRES AN X-RAY?

If it is accepted that not every head-injured patient can or should be X-rayed, there are great difficulties in deciding who to investigate in this way and who does not need it. The decision to X-ray any patient is based on clinical findings but, in contrast to patients with limb injuries, there are very few symptoms and signs which assist in making a positive diagnosis of a fracture of the skull vault. If a doctor feels that clinically there is no fracture, he will be right in 99% of cases (Royal College of Radiologists, 1983). However, almost every clinician has seen such a patient and has been convinced that there is no fracture and yet has X-rayed the patient for reassurance or some other reason and has been surprised to find a skull fracture. Unfortunately these unexpected fractures made up 23 out of 64 skull fractures in patients with uncomplicated head injuries (Royal College of Radiologists, 1981). Bruising of the scalp is difficult to see without shaving the hair, and skull fractures may occur when there are no external signs of injury. In one series, external evidence of trauma was found in only 72% of children with skull fractures (Harwood Nash, Hendrick and Hudson, 1971) (and in 16% of these the fracture was on the opposite side to the scalp injury). As many patients with head injuries may be amnesic for the event, it is also possible to have a skull fracture in the absence of either history or signs of injury. Reliance on clinical judgement is not adequate if all fractures are to be diagnosed and the threshold for doing skull X-rays needs to be low even though the incidence of fractures detected on skull X-rays is very small.

Guidelines

Because of the expense of radiology and the low yield of fractures, there has been much pressure to reduce the number of skull X-rays taken, and various studies have looked at factors which may predict a fracture. Unfortunately there are no invariable signs, and the best of the Royal College of Radiologists Working Party guidelines (1983) will miss 6% of currently diagnosed skull fractures. However, based on these guidelines, a group of neurosurgeons (1984) drew up a consensus as to who should be X-rayed following a head injury and a wider group reached similar conclusions at a conference organized by the DHSS (Anonymous, 1983). These guidelines are shown in Table 6.2. Others (Swann, MacMillan and Strang, 1981) feel that all patients with scalp lacerations should be X-rayed.

While neither these nor any guidelines can pick up all fractures, adhering to them will have the advantage that a doctor may avoid criticism or allegations of negligence if a fracture is missed.

Table 6.2 Criteria for skull X-ray after a recent head injury
(Anonymous, 1983)

Skull X-ray can be helpful but clinical judgement is necessary, and the following criteria will be refined by further experience. The presence of one or more of the following indicates a need for a skull X-ray in patients with a history of recent injury.

1. Loss of consciousness or amnesia at any time
2. Neurological symptoms or signs
3. Cerebrospinal fluid or blood from the nose or ear
4. Suspected penetrating injury or scalp bruising or swelling
5. Alcohol intoxication
6. Difficulty in assessing the patient (e.g. the young, epilepsy)

Note: simple scalp laceration is not a criterion for skull X-ray

FRACTURES MISSED ON X-RAY

Unfortunately, even when the decision has been made to X-ray a patient, skull fractures are still missed because the X-rays may be misinterpreted. The incidence of missed skull fractures in A & E departments is shown in Table 6.3 and varies between 9.2% (Gorman, 1987) and 60% in a small series with only 10 fractures (Vincent et al., 1988). A contributory factor may be that, in 27% of patients in one of these series, at least one of the X-ray films was inadequate (Swann, MacMillan and Strang, 1981). Radiologists too may miss skull fractures (Leaman et al., 1988). Junior medical staff working in A & E departments need more teaching on the interpretation of skull X-rays.

Table 6.3 Incidence of missed skull fractures

Author	Incidence of missed fractures
Gorman (1987)	9.2%
Swann, MacMillan and Strang (1981)	12.5%
Thillainayagam et al. (1987)	13.3%
Carew-McColl (1983)	30%
Royal College of Radiologists (1981)	30%
Vincent et al. (1988)	60%

THE CONSEQUENCES OF MISSING A SKULL FRACTURE

According to the figures of Mendelow et al. (1983) the incidence of intracranial haematoma in the orientated adult patient with a skull fracture (the type of patient who is likely to be discharged) is 1 in 32. With smaller numbers, the Royal College of Radiologists Working Party (1981) found that 4 patients developed intracranial haematomas out of 67 patients with skull fractures but otherwise uncomplicated injuries. Some of these patients may be admitted for other reasons and so the risk of an individual patient who has been discharged developing an intracranial haematoma is not high.

However, the consequences if a patient does develop a haematoma may be grave, depending on how rapidly any deterioration is detected and he returns to hospital, as the prognosis of an extradural haematoma is very dependent on the delay between the onset of deterioration and the evacuation of the haematoma (Mendelow et al., 1979).

COMPOUND DEPRESSED SKULL FRACTURES AND PENETRATING INJURIES

While the importance of diagnosing all linear skull fractures can be debated, there can be no argument about the importance of correctly diagnosing all compound depressed fractures and penetrating injuries of the skull because of the high risk of infection if they are not correctly diagnosed and managed. Fortunately they are uncommon, being found in 0.07% of skull X-rays in one series (Royal College of Radiologists, 1981) and 0.33% in another (Gorman, 1987). In a series of 359 compound depressed skull fractures (Jennett and Miller, 1972) the diagnosis was initially overlooked by hospital staff in 28 (many were not X-rayed) and 15 of these developed infections. Although these injuries are serious, there may be little initial brain injury, and 71% of the patients in whom the diagnosis was missed had lost consciousness only briefly or not at all. The fact that many patients were drunk made them harder to assess.

Suspicions of a depressed fracture should be raised by the history of being hit on the head with a small hard object, and exploration of all scalp wounds with a gloved finger before suturing them should reveal most depressed fractures. The X-ray appearances of depressed fractures, especially the significance of a line of increased density, should be sought and if there is any doubt a tangential X-ray of the suspected fracture will confirm the diagnosis.

Penetrating skull injuries are even less common and should be diagnosed on the history. The thinner the bone the more likely it is to be penetrated, and the thinnest part of the skull is the roof of the orbit. Penetrating injuries of the upper eyelid (e.g. with a pencil point) may be associated with penetration of the orbital roof, and these injuries are commonly overlooked (Guthkelch, 1960; Duffy and Bhandari, 1969; Foy and Scharr, 1980; Kirkby, 1986). In all cases of penetrating injuries of the upper eyelid, an X-ran should be done. If a fracture is seen, this is diagnostic of a cranial penetration (Duffy and Bhandari, 1969) but the absence of a fracture does not exclude it, and all these injuries should be taken very seriously. The other common site for penetrating injuries is the temporal bone.

COMPLICATIONS OF HEAD INJURY

Although uncommon, the most important complication (because it is so treatable) is intracranial haematoma, especially extradural haematoma. It is important not only to diagnose these but to do so early, as the longer treatment is delayed the worse is the outcome (Mendelow et al., 1979). For this reason, anybody at risk of an intracranial haematoma should be admitted to hospital for head injury observations. If large numbers of patients with negligible risk of complications are admitted, this is not only at great cost to the health service and patients, but the head injury observations are likely to be done less well and the rare complication may not be noted early (Chapter 5). If fewer patients at greater risk are admitted, complications should be detected earlier. The difficulty is in predicting those at risk, and this was recognized by Hippocrates several thousand years ago when he observed that there was no head injury so minor that it could be ignored. However, a recent study has shown that if a head injured adult is orientated and has no skull fracture the risk of developing an intracranial haematoma is only 1 in 5983 (Mendelow et al., 1983). This risk is surely acceptable (except to the rare person concerned) and so this group of patients can be discharged so long as they have someone to take care of them and there is no other problem (Group of Neurosurgeons, 1984). In a retrospective study of 100 patients with extradural haematomas and examined to test these criteria, it was found that three adults with extradural haematomas would have been discharged if these criteria were adhered to, but in two this was because the skull fracture was missed on X-ray (Sandeman and Cummins, 1986). Greater selection of patients for admission does necessitate accurate reading of skull X-rays.

Unfortunately children may develop extradural haematomas in the absence of skull fracture, and so any child with evidence of a significant head injury must be admitted even if there is no fracture.

Once admitted, the traditional management is that patients are regularly observed and investigated for intracranial haematoma by CT scan if their level of consciousness deteriorates or if they develop focal signs. Delayed diagnosis and misdiagnosis occur when this deterioration is either not observed or is attributed to another cause. The observations made should be easy to do without inter-observer variation and yet they should be sensitive enough to detect early deterioration. The Glasgow Coma Scale — a 12 point scale — is in use at most hospitals, but more sensitive scales have been devised (Price and Marsden, 1982) and might detect deterioration earlier, though their value is unproven.

While deterioration in conscious level is still a very important sign to be recognized as early as possible, it is known that haematomas may be seen on a CT scan before deterioration occurs. The aim should be to identify the group of patients at most risk from intracranial haematoma so that they can have a CT scan to enable the haematoma to be detected at this early stage. Clinical criteria to detect this group are somewhat insensitive but additional information provided by a computerized 'midliner' may lead to a better delineation of this 'at risk' group (Marsden and Price, 1988).

Many intracranial haematomas are misdiagnosed or diagnosed late, and this has been investigated by Galbraith (1976). In one group of patients with head injuries, 51 developed intracranial haematomas but 11 of these were not diagnosed until after necropsy. Six of these patients had been diagnosed clinically as having strokes and 5 had been thought to be drunk. In another group of 307 patients with intracranial haematomas referred to a neurosurgical unit, 111 had been deteriorating for more than 12 hours. Of these, 27 were initially thought to have had a stroke and 48 were thought to be drunk. In all, 29 of the 33 patients thought to have had a stroke had skull fractures, as did 41 of the 53 thought to have been drunk.

If a patient is thought to have had a stroke and is found to have a skull fracture, what he really has is a traumatic intracranial haematoma (Galbraith, 1976, 1987).

A high proportion of head injured patients have recently consumed alcohol (Swann, MacMillan and Strang, 1981), frequently in large amounts, and so the differentiation between the effects of the alcohol and the effects of the head injury is vital, but may be impossible clinically. This is further discussed in Chapter 5 but the only safe procedure at the time is to assume that any deterioration of conscious level is due to the head injury though, in retrospect, it may turn out that the patient was just drunk.

Chronic subdural haematomas also cause diagnostic difficulties (Brocklehurst, 1982), especially in patients with pre-existing neurological diseases (Harding, 1984) but this is not usually an A & E problem, and it will not be discussed further.

Table 6.4 How to differentiate skull fractures from other markings

Fractures	are sharply defined lines
	are straight but may have sudden changes in direction
	run across anatomical features such as sutures and blood vessels
	do not usually taper or branch
Sutures	occur in standard places
	are symmetrical
Blood vessels	are usually straight but may taper and branch
	are often bilateral
	may have a margin of cortical bone.

FALSE POSITIVE DIAGNOSIS OF SKULL FRACTURES

There is frequently confusion between fractures, sutures and vascular markings. Features to distinguish them are shown in Table 6.4. Confusion may also be caused by anatomical variants such as accessory sutures, especially in the occipital bone in children and the accessory midline frontal (metopic) suture.

The healing of skull fractures is very variable and, while some fractures may heal fully, others may still be visible several years later and may be confused with a recent injury. A history of a previous fracture may help, as will old X-rays. Although it has been pointed out above that some fractures may not be associated with external signs of injury or may be contralateral to such signs, if the history is of a blow to one side of the head and only to that one side and the fracture is on the other side, then the two are not related. Contra-coup brain injury is common but contracoup fractures do not occur.

A deep laceration of the scalp may show on X-ray as a radiolucency which can be confused with a fracture, but the lucency will correspond exactly with the wound if the wound is examined, no fracture can be palpated or seen and the lucency disappears if further X-rays are done after suturing the wound. Blood or dirt matted in the hair or even braided hair may cause a radiodense appearance which can be misdiagnosed as a depressed fracture (Mok, Gooll and Kreel, 1987). Examining the X-ray films against a bright light may show that the density is not confined to the bone margins but extends into the soft tissues and, if there is real confusion, tangential X-rays or further X-rays when blood has been cleaned away will be normal.

Bleeding from the ear following a head injury is usually caused by a temporal bone fracture but it may be caused by local injury to the external auditory meatus, especially in relation to fractures of the mandibular condyle.

FALSE POSITIVE DIAGNOSIS OF BRAIN INJURY

Other neurological diseases may cause confusion. The patient with pre-existing neurological signs, including pupillary changes from eye disease or eye drops, who falls and injures his head, may have his signs attributed to the injury. There is the frequent problem of deciding whether a patient has a fit resulting in a head injury or whether he falls, injuring his head, and then fits as a complication. Blows to the head are relatively common and so it is by no means rare for a patient with a stroke or other acute neurological problem to remember a minor head injury a few days earlier. The patient may also fall as a result of the stroke and so will be diagnosed as having traumatic intracranial haematoma. A CT scan will usually be needed.

Fits are a common acute complication of head injury and, if the clonic phase is minimal or not observed, the resulting deterioration in level of consciousness may be attributed to an intracranial haematoma. Usually the instant nature of the deterioration in consciousness suggests the diagnosis, and the patient should be given anticonvulsants and the level of consciousness should return to normal. If it does not, the patient should have a CT scan.

Following a minor head injury, many patients will have some weeks of headaches, dizziness, loss of concentration, tiredness and other vague symptoms — the post-traumatic syndrome (Kelly, 1981). It is very common for these patients to be referred back to A & E by their general practitioners with a diagnosis of '?Subdural'. A history that symptoms are getting better, a normal level of consciousness, full orientation and a normal neurological examination (save for occasional nystagmus) and a full explanation is usually enough to reassure patient, general practitioner and casualty officer, but better education of both doctors and patients about the likely course following a minor head injury might prevent these return visits.

Occasionally a patient with a severe head injury has its severity overestimated. Bilateral fixed dilated pupils is not a good prognostic sign, but patients who come in like this must not be misdiagnosed as having an irreversible brain injury, as the significant number of patients (especially children) can make a good recovery from this.

REFERENCES

Anonymous (1983) Guidelines for the management of patients with recent head injury. In *The Management of Acute Head Injury.* Fenton Lewis A. (ed.), London, Dept. of Health and Social Security, p. 3.

Brocklehurst G. (1982) Diagnoses not to be missed: subdural haematoma. *Br. J. Hosp. Med.*, **27**, 170–4.

Carew-McColl M. (1983) Radiological interpretation in an accident and emergency department. *Br. J. Clin. Pract.*, **37**, 375–7.

Duffy G.P. and Bhandari Y.S. (1969) Intracranial complications following transorbital penetrating injuries. *Br. J. Surg.*, **56**, 685–8.

Evans K.T. (1977) The radiologist's dilemma. *Br. J. Radiol.*, **50**, 299–301.

Foy P. and Scharr M. (1980) Cerebral abscesses in children after pencil tip injuries. *Lancet*, **ii**, 662–3.

Fullarton G.M., McEwen C.J., MacMillan R. et al. (1987) An evaluation of open scalp wounds. *Arch. Emerg. Med.*, **4**, 11–16.

Galbraith S. (1976) Misdiagnosis and delayed diagnosis in traumatic intracranial haematoma. *Br. Med. J.*, **1**, 1438–9.

Galbraith S. (1987) Head injuries in the elderly. *Br. Med. J.*, **294**, 325.

Gorman D.F. (1987) The utility of post-traumatic skull X-rays. *Arch. Emerg. Med.*, **4**, 141–50.

Group of Neurosurgeons (1984) Guidelines for initial management after head injury in adults. *Br. Med. J.*, **288**, 983–5.

Guthkelch A.N. (1960) Apparently trivial wounds of the eyelids with intracranial damage. *Br. Med. J.*, **2**, 842–4.

Harding A.E. (1984) Subdural haematoma in two patients with chronic neurological disorders. *Br. Med. J.*, **288**, 1986–7.

Harwood Nash D.C., Hendrick E.B. and Hudson A.R. (1971) The significance of skull fractures in children: a study of 1187 patients. *Radiology*, **101**, 151–5.

Jennett B. (1987) Skull X-rays after minor head injuries. *Arch. Emerg. Med.*, **4**, 133–5.

Jennett B. and Miller J.D. (1972) Infection after depressed fracture of the skull. *J. Neurosurg.*, **36**, 333–9.

Kelly R. (1981) The post-traumatic syndrome. *J. Roy. Soc. Med.*, **74**, 242–4.

Kirkby G.R. (1986) Penetrating orbitocranial injury with a snooker cue. *Br. Med. J.*, **293**, 1646.

Leaman A.M., Gorman D.F., Danher J. et al. (1988) Skull X-rays after trauma: are both laterals necessary? *Arch. Emerg. Med.*, **5**, 18–20.

Marsden A.K. and Price D.J. (1988) The minor head injury. *Arch. Emerg. Med.*, **5**, 1–3.

Mendelow A.D., Karma M.Z., Paul K.S. et al. (1979) Extradural haematoma: effect of delayed treatment. *Br. Med. J.*, **1**, 1240–2.

Mendelow A.D., Teasdale G., Jennett B. et al. (1983) Risks of intracranial haematoma in head injured adults. *Br. Med. J.*, **287**, 1173–6.

Mok D.W.H., Gooll C.J. and Kreel L. (1987) Pseudofractures of the skull. *Br. J. Acc. Emerg. Med.*, **2** June, 10–13.

Price D.J. and Marsden A.K. (1982) A practical scale for monitoring head injuries. In *Care of the Acutely Ill and Injured*. Wilson D.H. and Marsden A.K. (ed.), Chichester, Wiley, pp. 353–8.

Royal College of Radiologists Working Party (1980) A study of the utilisation of skull radiography in accident and emergency departments in the U.K. *Lancet*, **ii**, 1234–7.

Royal College of Radiologists Working Party (1981) Costs and benefits of skull radiography for head injury. *Lancet,* **ii,** 791–5.

Royal College of Radiologists Working Party (1983) Patient selection for skull radiography in uncomplicated head injury. *Lancet,* **i,** 115–8.

Sandeman D.R. and Cummins B.C. (1986) The provenance of extradural haematomas. *Br. Med. J.,* **292,** 522–3.

Swann I.J., MacMillan R. and Strang I. (1981) Head injuries at an inner city accident and emergency department. *Injury,* **12,** 274–8.

Thillainayagam K., Macmillan R., Mendelow A.D. et al. (1987) How accurately are fractures of the skull diagnosed in an accident and emergency department? *Injury,* **18,** 319–21.

Vincent C.A., Driscoll P.A., Audley R.J. et al. (1988) Accuracy of detection of radiographic abnormalities by junior doctors. *Arch. Emerg. Med.,* **5,** 101–9.

Waldron J. and Hurley S.E.J. (1988) Temporal bone fractures: a clinical diagnosis. *Arch. Emerg. Med.,* **5,** 146–50.

Webber R.L. and Folio J. (1976) Radiographic detectability of occipital and temporal-parietal fractures in cadaver heads. *J. Trauma,* **16,** 115–24.

7   Spinal injuries

INTRODUCTION

Many injuries, if missed, may cause pain, inconvenience and delay in commencing treatment, which may or may not influence the prognosis. However, to miss a spinal injury may be to cause tragedy if a neurologically intact patient is rendered paraplegic or tetraplegic or if a patient with neurological damage is made worse.

INCIDENCE OF MISSED SPINAL INJURY

Several series have looked at missed spinal injuries, and the incidence varies from series to series, depending on the exact injury looked at. In a series of patients with spinal cord injuries, the injury was missed in 4.3% of patients (Ravichandran and Silver, 1982), but the incidence of missed fractures and dislocations is much higher. In a series of injuries described from spinal injuries units, 22.9% of cervical spine injuries and 4.9% of thoracodorsal injuries were missed initially (Reid et al., 1987), as were 40% of patients with facet joint dislocations who sought medical help (Braakman and Vinken, 1968) and 42% of the fractures in patients with tetraplegia due to hyperextension injuries (McMillan and Silver, 1987). Two-thirds of dislocations at the cervicothoracic junction were not properly diagnosed on admission in another series (Evans, 1983). In a radiological study, only 22% of cervical spine injuries were correctly diagnosed (Annis et al., 1987).

WHY ARE INJURIES MISSED?

A review shows that errors are made at all the stages of the diagnostic process, as detailed in Chapter 2, and in many cases there is more than one factor involved.

History

The patient's inability to give a history or to describe symptoms is a major cause of problems. The main reason for this is a diminished level of consciousness due to a head injury, which is frequently associated with a spinal injury, and in these circumstances the spinal injury is often missed (Scher, 1981; Ravichandran and Silver, 1982; Evans, 1983; Shalley and Cross, 1984). This is further discussed in Chapter 22.

Even if a patient is able to give an account of himself, a failure to take enough history to understand the mechanism and forces involved in the injury is also a major contributory cause of missed injuries (Ravichandran and Silver, 1982).

Examination

If a patient presents with an isolated spinal injury, failure to examine the spine and the nervous system would amount to negligence, but parts of the examination may be omitted. Thus a torticollis may be assumed to be due to muscle spasm, but this needs to be looked for as, in the absence of sternomastoid spasm, it is likely to be due to a unilateral facet joint dislocation (Ross et al., 1987).

Misdiagnosis of spinal injuries due to failures in examination is more likely to occur in the patient with multiple injuries (Ravichandran and Silver, 1982), when the patient may not be turned to examine the spine, priapism and absence of intercostal breathing may be overlooked as pointers to spinal injury, and weakness may be difficult to assess because of limb injuries. If a patient requires intubation and ventilation because of a head or chest injury, it is impossible to test for neurological deficit once the patient is paralysed. It is therefore vital that a brief neurological assessment is done before muscle relaxants are given, or the diagnosis of paraplegia may be missed. This is further discussed in Chapter 22.

Failure to X-ray

Some spinal injuries are missed for this reason (Braakman and Vinken, 1968; Ravichandran and Silver, 1982; Evans, 1983; Reid et al., 1987) but this is usually secondary to failures of history taking and examination and to failure to X-ray the cervical spine routinely in all cases of head injury.

The circumstances in which a patient injures himself should not be allowed to influence a doctor's judgement, as this is a factor in some missed spinal injuries (Ravichandran and Silver, 1982).

X-ray interpretation

The major cause of missing spinal injuries, especially cervical spinal injuries, is problems with X-rays and their interpretation.

The cervical spine consists of seven vertebrae and, unless an X-ray shows all seven and the top of the first thoracic vertebra, it is not an X-ray of the cervical spine but it is an X-ray of part of the spine. There may be an injury in the part not X-rayed, and this will be missed. The commonest problem with cervical spine X-rays is failure to show the cervicodorsal junction (Braakman and Vinken, 1968; Ravichandran and Silver, 1982; Evans, 1983; Annis et al., 1987) which is a common site for injuries. In one series, only 57% of lateral cervical spine X-rays showed this, though 24% of the injuries were at this site (Annis et al., 1987). An open mouth view to demonstrate the odontoid and the cervicocranial junction may also be difficult to obtain if the patient is uncooperative, and the same study (Annis et al., 1987) showed that this was available in only 67% of 703 cervical spine X-rays. X-rays may be inadequate or of poor quality for other reasons too (Chapter 3). Inadequate cervical spine X-rays have been found to constitute 53% (Ravichandran and Silver, 1982), 42% (Bryan, 1988) and 25.9% (Ross et al., 1987) of a series of spinal X-rays and missed spinal fractures.

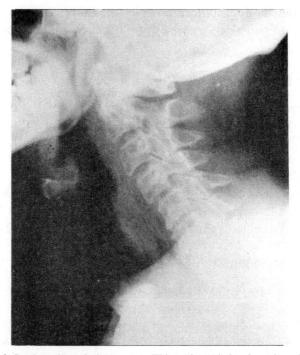

Figure 7.1 Look at the soft tissues, too. This patient tried to hang herself. An X-ray was taken to exclude bony injury and shows no bony injury (but the C7/T1 junction is not shown). However, there is surgical emphysema in the neck indicating (in this case) a fractured larynx.

Unfortunately, even if adequate, cervical spine X-rays are easily misinterpreted (Scher, 1981; Ravichandran and Silver, 1982) and in one series already mentioned (Annis et al., 1987) only 2 of 6 subluxations and 3 out of 17 fractures were diagnosed by the casualty officers.

Of particular importance are the subtle changes of anterior subluxation of the cervical spine (Evans, 1976; Webb et al., 1976) which are easily missed. These are listed in Table 7.1. If there is doubt about the diagnosis of this injury, flexion/extension neck X-rays can be performed if the patient is fully conscious.

Table 7.1 Subtle X-ray changes which may indicate a severe injury

Hyperflexion injuries
Kyphotic angulation of the contour of the curve of the cervical spine localized to one disc space
Widening of the prevertebral soft tissue
Widening of the interspinous space and divergence of the spinous processes
Narrowing of the disc space anteriorly

Hyperextension injuries
Avulsion fracture of the anterior surface of the vertebral body or fracture of an anterior osteophyte
Fracture of a spinous process
Widening of the disc space

In addition to the bony abnormalities on an X-ray, attention must also be directed to the soft tissues, as soft-tissue swelling may be an important sign of injury, drawing attention to a bony injury missed at first glance or to an injury not visible on initial films (Gopalakrishnan and El Masri, 1986).

X-rays are much more difficult to interpret if a patient has severe degenerative changes in the neck or osteoporotic changes in the lumbar spine.

Minor crush fractures of the lumbar spine may be missed if the inexperienced casualty officer is unaware of what he is looking for. Crush fractures of the lower thoracic spine may be overlooked if an X-ray of the lumbar spine is requested, and only the lumbar vertebrae are examined rather than every bone visible.

Fractures of the transverse processes of the lumbar spine may be difficult to see because of overlying bowel gas.

INJURIES IN THE PRESENCE OF A NORMAL X-RAY

Even if the cervical spine X-ray is normal, the patient may still have serious spinal or cord injury. These patients fall into two categories.

In the first are those with hyperflexion injuries, with ligamentous rupture and instability but no subluxation or dislocation, as the bony alignment is held by muscle spasm. If a patient has severe neck pain following an injury, this must be taken seriously and, if the initial X-rays are adequate and are normal, then stress (flexion/extension) X-rays should be performed to exclude instability (Spencer and Birtcliffe, 1985; Plunkett, Redmond and Billsborough, 1987). These must be done actively by the patient within the limits of his pain. They should not be attempted unless the patient is fully conscious and alert and, under no circumstances, should the head be moved passively.

The second group are usually middle-aged or elderly patients with cervical spondylosis, who suffer a hyperextension neck injury and who develop a central cord syndrome with the neurological deficit involving the arms more than the legs and with bladder involvement. This deficit may initially be missed, especially if the patient is drunk or smells of alcohol, when he may be diagnosed as drunk (Hardy, 1977; Maxted and Dowd, 1982).

PRE-EXISTING DISEASES

Pre-existing disease may make diagnosis more difficult. A fused cervical spine, due to ankylosing spondylitis or ankylosing vertebral hyperostosis, may fracture with minimal trauma that would not be expected to injure a normal neck (Grisolia, Bell and Peltier, 1967; Hunter and Dubo, 1978; Corke, 1981). In addition, X-rays may be difficult to do and interpret because of deformity and osteoporosis. Patients at risk of pathological fractures from whatever cause may also fracture their spines with minimal trauma.

Patients with pre-existing neurological diseases, who injure their necks and who are found to have neurological signs, may have these signs misinterpreted as being due to a progression of the disease rather than to the injury (Ravichandran and Silver, 1982).

MORE THAN ONE SPINAL INJURY

It is not rare for a patient with one spinal fracture to have a second spinal injury (7.8% in one series (Korres et al., 1981), in which case one of the fractures may be missed (Korres et al., 1981; Reid et al., 1987).

FALSE POSITIVES

Congenital abnormalities of the spine, including spina bifida occulta, fused vertebrae, hemivertebrae, etc. are common and may mystify inexperienced doctors. They are not, however, usually misdiagnosed as injuries, but pre-exisiting spondylolisthesis, spondylosis and atlanto-axial subluxation may cause diagnostic difficulties. In the open mouth view of the odontoid process, the teeth are often superimposed on the odontoid, which may be confused with fracture. Vertebral collapse due to osteoporosis may be difficult to age, and so previous crush fractures of the lumbar spine may be diagnosed as new injuries. Congenital abnormalities of the transverse processes of the lumbar spine are not uncommon and may be misdiagnosed as fractures, as may overlying bowel gas shadows.

A patient with a back injury of any severity may be more comfortable lying flat in bed but, in this position, many patients are unable to pass urine. The unwary doctor may diagnose a paraplegia but, if sacral sensation is intact and anal tone is normal, then the bladder dysfunction is not neurological.

Unrecognized bilateral shoulder dislocation may be misdiagnosed as a central cord syndrome, and unrecognized bilateral fractured neck of femur may be misdiagnosed as a paraplegia (Chapter 22).

Rarely paraplegia may be hysterical (Baker and Silver, 1987). This is clearly a dangerous diagnosis to make initially, but should be considered in the patient with motor paralysis in association with normal muscle tone and reflexes and non-anatomical sensory loss.

Practical points

● Have a low threshold for X-raying the cervical spine following injury. In particular, *always* X-ray the cervical spine in *all* unconscious head injuries and in any other patient following on injury and who it is difficult to assess, e.g. because of alcohol. Always X-ray the neck of patients with ankylosing spondylitis and those at risk of metastases, no matter how minimal the trauma.

- X-ray the whole spine of patients with multiple injuries.
- If you cannot see the top of T1, you have not got an X-ray of the cervical spine. Repeat it with downward traction on the arms or ask for a swimmer's view. If you still cannot see it, ask advice, as tomograms or CT scanning may be required.
- Beware the patient with torticollis but no muscle spasm. This may represent a facet joint dislocation.
- If a patient has severe neck pain but normal X-rays, flexion/extension X-rays should be done if the patient is fully conscious and alert. If not, treat the patient as for an injury until it is safe to do them.
- Beware the drunk who falls and has a hyperextension injury to the neck demonstrated by bruising of the forehead. He may have a central cord syndrome.

REFERENCES

Annis J.A.D., Finlay D.B.L., Allen M.J. et al. (1987) A review of cervical spine radiographs in casualty patients. *Br. J. Radiol.*, **60**, 1059–61.

Baker J.H.E. and Silver J.R. (1987) Hysterical paraplegia. *J. Neurol. Neurosurg. Psychiatry,* **50**, 375–82.

Braakman R. and Vinken P.J. (1968) Old luxations of the lower cervical spine. *J. Bone Jt Surg.,* **50B**, 52–60.

Bryan A.S. (1988) A review of cervical spine X-rays from a casualty department. *J. R. Coll. Surg. Edinb.,* **33**, 143–5.

Corke C.F. (1981) Spinal fracture and paraplegia after minimal trauma in a patient with ankylosing vertebral hyperostosis. *Br. Med. J.,* **282**, 2035.

Evans D.K. (1976) Anterior cervical subluxation. *J. Bone Jt Surg.,* **58B**, 318–21.

Evans D.K. (1983) Dislocations at the cervicothoracic junction. *J. Bone Jt Surg.,* **65B**, 124–7.

Gopalakrishnan K.C. and El Masri W. (1986) Prevertebral soft tissue shadow widening — an important sign of cervical spinal injury. *Injury,* **17**, 125–8.

Grisolia A., Bell R.L. and Peltier L.F. (1967) Fractures and dislocations of the spine complicating ankylosing spondylitis. *J. Bone Jt Surg.,* **49A**, 339–44.

SPINAL INJURIES

Hardy A.G. (1977) Cervical spinal cord injury without bony injury. *Paraplegia,* **14,** 296–305.

Hunter T. and Dubo H. (1978) Spinal fractures complicating ankylosing spondylitis. *Ann. Int. Med.,* **88,** 546–9.

Korres D.S., Katsaros A., Pantazopoulos T. et al. (1981) Double or multiple level fractures of the spine. *Injury,* **13,** 147–52.

McMillan B.S. and Silver J.R. (1987) Extension injuries to the cervical spine resulting in tetraplegia. *Injury,* **18,** 224–33.

Maxted M.J. and Dowd G.S.E. (1982) Acute central cord syndrome without bony injury. *Injury,* **14,** 103–6.

Plunkett P.K., Redmond A.D. and Billsborough S.H. (1987) Cervical subluxation: a deceptive soft tissue injury. *J. R. Soc. Med.,* **80,** 46–7.

Ravichandran G. and Silver J.R. (1982) Missed injuries of the spinal cord. *Br. Med. J.,* **284,** 953–6.

Ravichandran G. and Silver J.R. (1984) Recognition of spinal cord injury. *Hospital Update,* Jan. 77–86.

Reid D.C., Henderson R., Saboe L. et al. (1987) Etiology and clinical course of missed spine fractures. *J. Trauma,* **27,** 980–6.

Ross S.E., Schwab W., David E.T. et al. (1987) Clearing the cervical spine: initial radiologic evaluation. *J. Trauma,* **27,** 1055–60.

Scher A.T. (1981) Unrecognised fractures and dislocations of the cervical spine. *Paraplegia,* **19,** 25–30.

Shalley M.J. and Cross A.B. (1984) Which patients are likely to die in an accident and emergency department? *Br. Med. J.,* **289,** 419–21.

Spencer J.D. and Birtcliffe I.W.L. (1985) Injury to the cervical spine after a game of British Bulldog. *Br. Med. J.,* **290,** 1888–9.

Webb J.K., Broughton R.B.K., McSweeney T. et al. (1976) Hidden flexion injury of the cervical spine. *J. Bone Jt Surg.,* **58B,** 322–7.

8   Facial injuries

FRACTURED ZYGOMA AND ORBITAL FLOOR

The fractured zygoma is a commonly missed fracture (Wardrope and Chennells, 1985).

It may be a difficult diagnosis to make clinically as soft tissue swelling may obscure any deformity and, if it causes any difficulty with eye opening, will also hide any diplopia. X-rays, too, may be difficult to interpret because of soft tissue swelling. X-rays must be of good quality and taken PA rather than AP. These cannot usually be done on an A & E trolley and will necessitate moving the patient. There is no point in trying to get X-rays of diagnostic quality on an uncooperative drunk, but it is better to wait and do them when the patient is sober.

Standard X-rays may not show fractures, though pointers, such as a fluid level or obscurity of the antrum and surgical emphysema of the orbit, should also be looked for. However, other types of X-rays may reveal fractures not seen on standard views (Evans, 1985). For this reason, any patient with good clinical evidence of a fracture (Table 8.1), should be referred for a specialist opinion, even if no fracture is seen on initial X-rays.

Table 8.1 Clinical signs of fractured zygoma and orbital floor

---

Black eye
Deformity (may be obscured by soft tissue swelling)
'Step' orbital rim
Tenderness, including tenderness of the zygomaticofrontal suture
Diplopia (especially on upward gaze)
Limitation of upward gaze
Numbness of cheek (due to involvement of infra-orbital nerve) and of upper teeth
Surgical emphysema of the orbit
Lateral subconjuctival haemorrhage without posterior limit

Fractures of the orbital floor, including blow-out fractures, may also have normal X-rays. Some faciomaxillary surgeons like to investigate all patients with suspected fractures of the zygoma with tomography to exclude orbital floor injury, but the presence of limitation of, or diplopia on, upward gaze or the presence of a soft-tissue swelling in the roof of the antrum on facial X-rays makes referral for tomography essential (Figure 8.1).

Displaced fractures of the zygomatic arch may impinge on the coronoid process of the mandible, thus limiting jaw movements and so leading the casualty officer to suspect a mandibular injury rather than a zygomatic injury.

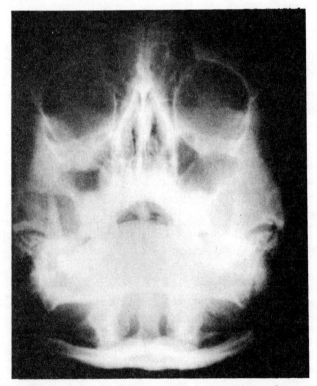

Figure 8.1 Blow-out fracture of the orbit. No bony injury is seen but note the soft-tissue swelling in the roof of the right antrum and the probable fluid level. This patient needs tomograms of the orbital floor.

FRACTURED MANDIBLE

Soft-tissue injuries of the face are rightly considered important, but underlying fractures should not be overlooked (Myall, Sandor and Gregory, 1987). Some mandibular fractures may be difficult to demonstrate radiologically, especially fractures of the condyles and fractures in the midline, which accounts for the many different X-rays which may be taken (Table 8.2). If the inexperienced casualty officer feels that the patient has a fracture clinically but cannot see it on standard X-rays, he should seek advice.

Table 8.2 Mandibular X-rays

AP
Lateral
Left and right obliques
Submentovertical (to show midline)
Modified Towne's view (to show condyles)
Orthopantomogram
Intra-oral dental X-rays
TM joint views

As the posterior wall of the temporomandibular joint is also the anterior wall of the external auditory meatus, injuries to the condyle of the mandible may cause trauma to the external ear which results in bleeding from the ear. This may be misdiagnosed as being due to a fractured base of skull.

DISLOCATION OF THE TEMPOROMANDIBULAR JOINT

This may be overlooked, especially in patients with other medical problems (Wright, 1985).

NASAL INJURIES

The examination of the nose following trauma must include examining the airway and looking into the nostrils, as otherwise traumatic septal deviation and septal haematoma will be missed. Nasal bone fractures may also commonly be overdiagnosed (Gleadhill, Thompson and Simms, 1987) and missed (de Lacey et al., 1977) on X-ray.

EYE INJURIES

Blunt and perforating injuries of the eye may be overlooked in patients with other injuries, and this worsens the prognosis (Soni and Eustace, 1972). In any patient with lacerations of the eyelid, the eye itself should be examined (if necessary using local anaesthetic and retractors) for diminished visual acuity, haemorrhage, deformity of the pupil and haziness of the media.

Penetrating injuries of the eyelids causing penetration of the anterior cranial fossa have been discussed in Chapter 6. Penetrating injuries of the eye itself may also do this (Hakin, 1988).

Intra-ocular foreign bodies are discussed in Chapter 20.

OTHER SOFT-TISSUE FACIAL INJURIES

Depending on the site, facial lacerations may divide tear ducts, parotid duct or facial nerve. Advice should be sought for all deep facial lacerations.

REFERENCES
Evans R. (1985) Rotational panoramic zonography (Equipment review). *Arch. Emerg. Med.*, **2**, 97–103.

Gleadhill D.N.S., Thompson J.Y. and Simms P. (1987) Can more efficient use be made of X-ray examinations in the accident and emergency department? *Br. Med. J.*, **294**, 943–7.

Hakin K.B. (1988) More than meets the eye. *Br. Med. J.*, **296**, 429–30.

de Lacey G.J., Wignall B.K., Hussein S. et al. (1977) The radiology of nasal injuries: problems of interpretation and clinical relevance. *Br. J. Radiol.*, **50**, 412–4.

Myall R.W.T., Sandor G.K.B. and Gregory C.E.B. (1987) Are you overlooking fractures of the mandibular condyle? *Paediatrics*, **79**, 639–41.

Soni K.G. and Eustace P. (1972) Missed ocular perforations after road traffic accidents. *Injury*, **4**, 79–80.

Wardrope J. and Chennells P.M. (1985) Should all casualty radiographs be reviewed? *Br. Med. J.*, **290**, 1638–40.

Wright A.J. (1985) An unusual but easily treatable cause of dysphagia and dysarthria complicating stroke. *Br. Med. J.*, **291**, 1412–13.

9   Chest injuries

INTRODUCTION

Keen (1984) states that it is probable that 'most fatal mistakes in the management of chest injuries result from errors in diagnosis or incomplete diagnosis'. The early diagnosis of chest injuries and their treatment is important, not just to prevent avoidable deaths from the injuries themselves, but also because the correct management of extrathoracic injuries (especially head injuries) depends on the urgent correction of hypoxia and hypercarbia, and the correct management of an associated chest injury is a very important step towards this.

However, the diagnosis of chest injuries is not always easy, as is shown by a paper describing missed and delayed diagnoses in 90 patients with major blunt chest injuries (Blair, Topuzlu and Davis, 1971). The results of this are summarized in Table 9.1.

Table 9.1 Missed diagnoses in blunt chest injury. Data from Blair, Topuzlu and Davis, 1971

Condition	Number of patients	Number missed in emergency room or on admission
Flail chest	80	25
Fracture or dislocation of sternum	8	3
Ruptured diaphragm	3	3
Haemopericardium	2	2
Ruptured bronchus	1	1
Myocardial contusion	20	20

In addition only 2 out of 8 tension pneumothoraces were diagnosed clinically

RIB FRACTURES

About a third of patients with rib fractures will have no fracture visible on an AP or PA chest X-ray (Danher, Eyes and Kumar, 1984) and, in the same series, one patient had five rib fractures and a normal chest X-ray. To diagnose all rib fractures, it is therefore necessary to do oblique rib views and possibly other X-rays (e.g. to show the lower ribs). Despite this, the authors of the paper mentioned above concluded that routine oblique rib X-rays are unnecessary, and others agree (de Lacey, 1976). Is it important to diagnose rib fractures?

The strict answer is 'No', as there is no specific treatment for a fractured rib, and the management of a chest wall injury is the management of pain, of any underlying lung injury and of any complication. There is no direct relationship between rib fractures and complications, and many people who die of chest injuries do so without a single fracture.

However, a practical view (though unproven) is that a rib fracture will cause more pain than bruising of the chest wall and this pain may persist for longer. Patients with several fractures will have more pain still and so will need more analgesia and must be more at risk of developing complications such as haemothorax or chest infections. Many hospitals, therefore, operate policies to admit all patients with two or more rib fractures for chest physiotherapy and analgesia (which may need intercostal nerve blocks for which knowledge of rib fractures is necessary). In addition, there is an association between displaced fractures of the first rib and brachial plexus and subclavian artery injuries, and an association between lower rib fractures and injuries to the liver, spleen and kidney.

Thus, if from the history and the examination, there is the possibility of more than one rib fracture, it is important that these all be diagnosed in the acutely injured patient. Therefore these patients should have oblique rib X-rays (though they may have a low priority if a patient has other injuries). There is less need to confirm rib fractures radiologically in a patient who presents several days later and who clearly has no complication.

FLAIL CHEST

This is a clinical diagnosis based on observing abnormal chest movement as, although it may be diagnosed on a chest X-ray if one sees ribs fractured in two places, the X-ray is often normal if the fractures are through the costal cartilages rather than ribs. Occasionally a flail chest may not be apparent on admission if abnormal movement is prevented by muscle spasm but it may become obvious later. Usually it is missed because it is not looked for or observed.

STERNAL INJURIES

These require a lateral X-ray of the sternum for diagnosis. However, as even displaced fractures need no immediate treatment, this X-ray should wait until the patient's condition is stable.

SCAPULAR FRACTURES

Scapular fractures may be associated with significant chest wall injuries and, although the fracture is usually visible on the chest X-ray, it may be missed (Harris and Harris, 1988). On occasions, the scapula may not be visible either because it is not included on the chest X-ray or because it is obscured by superimposed structures, including the X-ray label (Harris and Harris). The possibility of scapular fracture should be considered and, if clinically suspected, specific scapular X-rays should be requested (Chapter 11).

PNEUMOTHORAX

A tension pneumothorax is easily diagnosed on an X-ray but the delay in getting an X-ray may be life threatening. It should therefore be diagnosed and treated on its clinical features (shortness of breath, diminished air entry and mediastinal shift) but it is often missed clinically (Blair, Topuzlu and Davis, 1971).

Other pneumothoraces are usually easily seen on an erect chest X-ray, though smaller ones are often missed, almost always because the X-ray has not been looked at carefully enough. However, if a patient has severe surgical emphysema of the chest wall, the radiological appearances of this may obscure the lung markings and make it impossible to diagnose either clinically or on a chest X-ray. If this occurs, it may be necessary to assume that there is a pneumothorax and to insert a chest drain without radiological proof.

If it is necessary for the patient to remain lying down because of other injuries, a supine chest X-ray will not give nearly as much information as an erect X-ray, and pneumothoraces (and haemothoraces) are easily missed (Cooke and Cooke, 1987; Cummin, Smith and Wilson, 1987). Although the radiological features of a pneumothorax on a supine X-ray have been described (Cooke and Cooke, 1987; Cummin, Smith and Wilson, 1987) (Table 9.1), it is safer to obtain a horizontal beam decubitus X-ray with the patient lying on the unaffected side, which will confirm the diagnosis. Pneumothoraces are also easily diagnosed on a CT scan and so, if a patient with multiple injuries is having a CT scan of some other part of the body (e.g. the head), it may be wise to do one or more cuts of the chest in addition, to exclude pneumothorax.

Table 9.1 Radiological signs of a pneumothorax in a supine patient (Cummin, Smith and Wilson, 1987)

1. Relative transradiancy of the lower chest and upper quadrant of the abdomen
2. Deepening of the lateral costophrenic sulcus
3. Appearance of the anterior costophrenic sulcus as an oblique interface extending downwards and outwards across the diaphragm, giving a double diaphragm appearance
4. Sharp delineation of the diaphragm and cardiac border with apical pericardial fat pads sometimes appearing as lobulated discrete opacities
5. A vertical line on the right just inside and parallel to the chest wall, caused by retraction of the middle lobe from the chest wall

It is of great importance that pneumothoraces be correctly diagnosed in traumatized patients as, if the patient requires positive pressure ventilation either for an anaesthetic or as a treatment for head or chest injuries, then any pneumothorax should be drained to prevent it increasing in size.

It should be noted that 10% of patients with a penetrating chest injury who have a normal chest X-ray will develop a haemothorax or pneumothorax later (Weigelt et al., 1982). These patients should be observed and re-X-rayed after 6 hours if this is not to be missed.

DIAPHRAGMATIC HERNIA

This may result from both penetrating and closed trauma and is frequently missed (Blair, Topuzlu and Davis, 1971; Bryer et al., 1978; Brearley and Tubbs, 1980; Carter, 1987; Feliciano et al., 1987).

The most common reason for missing it is misinterpretation of the chest X-ray which (though it may not always be diagnostic) is almost always abnormal. Difficulties occur particularly when it is associated with a haemothorax or lung contusion. Most cases are associated with intra-abdominal injury and so, even if missed pre-operatively, the diagnosis should be made at laparotomy, though it can be missed even then (Feliciano et al., 1987). Numerous ways of trying to confirm the diagnosis have been recommended including CT, ultrasound, gastro-intestinal contrast X-rays, fluoroscopy, laparoscopy and thoracoscopy, but the important thing is to suspect it clinically and on a plain chest X-ray, when further advice can be sought.

BLUNT CARDIAC INJURIES

Myocardial contusion

The diagnostic criteria for myocardial contusion are ill defined. Its diagnosis depends clinically on serial ECG changes and the development of complications such as arrhythmias, conduction disturbances and heart failure. Serum cardiac enzyme levels will be raised and tests of cardiac function, such as isotope scans, may be abnormal (Bancewizc and Yates, 1983). All patients with severe blunt chest injuries should have a 12-lead ECG on admission and then serially and should undergo cardiac monitoring.

Cardiac tamponade

This should be suspected in the patient who is shocked (without evidence of blood loss), cyanosed and dyspnoeic. A chest X-ray may be normal but the diagnosis is given by finding distended neck veins and confirmed by finding a raised central venous pressure.

Other injuries

Other cardiac injuries, such as septal defects or valve injuries, are rare but must be diagnosed early. They should be suspected in the patient (without any past history) who is noted to have a heart murmur or who develops cardiac failure.

RUPTURED AORTA

This is an easily and frequently missed injury. Its diagnosis depends on a high index of suspicion, an awareness of the radiological features listed in Table 9.2 and early use of angiography or CT scanning.

Table 9.2 Radiological signs of a ruptured thoracic aorta
(Ettinger, Hassan and Northup, 1983)

1. Widened mediastinum
2. Deviation of trachea to the right
3. Blurring or distortion of aortic contour
4. Opacification of space between the left pulmonary artery and the aorta
5. Obliteration of the medial border of the left upper lobe
6. Depression of the left main bronchus below 40°
7. Deviation of oesophagus (nasogastric tube) to right

PENETRATING INJURIES

Penetrating injuries, by virtue of leaving a wound, are usually easily diagnosed (but don't forget to look at the back). However, patients may have several stab wounds and it is possible for serious injuries to be overlooked if all one's attention is directed towards one injury. Any wound which could have involved the mediastinum should be assumed to have done so until proved otherwise. The dome of the diaphragm may rise to the fourth intercostal space during expiration, and so stab wounds at this level or below may cause an abdominal injury which will be missed if the diagnosis is not considered (Feliciano et al., 1984). Likewise, stab wounds of the abdominal wall may involve the thoracic cavity.

Practical points

● Many patients with chest injuries may have a normal chest X-ray initially and diagnosis depends on clinical signs, a high index of suspicion, other investigations and serial chest X-rays.

● All chest X-rays done for trauma should be taken erect if possible. If this is not possible, do horizontal beam decubitus X-rays with the patient lying first on one side and then on the other.

REFERENCES

Bancewizc J. and Yates D. (1983) Blunt injury to the heart. *Br. Med. J.,* **286,** 497–8.

Blair E., Topuzlu C. and Davis J.H. (1971) Delayed or missed diagnosis in blunt chest injury. *J. Trauma,* **11,** 129–45.

Brearley S. and Tubbs N. (1980) Rupture of the diaphragm in blunt injuries of the trunk. *Injury,* **12,** 480–4.

Bryer J.V., Hegarty M.M., Howe C. et al. (1978) Traumatic diaphragmatic hernia. *Br. J. Surg.,* **65,** 69–73.

Carter J.W. (1987) Diaphragmatic trauma in Southern Saskatchewan – an 11-year review. *J. Trauma,* **27,** 987–93.

Cooke D.A.P. and Cooke J.C. (1987) The supine pneumothorax. *Ann. R. Coll. Surg. Engl.,* **69,** 130–4.

Cummin A.R.C., Smith M.J. and Wilson A.G. (1987) Pneumothorax in the supine patient. *Br. Med. J.,* **295,** 591–2.

Danher J., Eyes B.E. and Kumar K. (1984) Oblique rib views after blunt chest trauma: an unnecessary routine? *Br. Med. J.,* **289,** 1271.

de Lacey G. (1976) Clinical and economic aspects of the use of X-rays in the accident and emergency department. *Proc. R. Soc. Med.,* **69,** 758–9.

Ettinger M.C., Hassan M. and Northup H.M. (1983) The radiological diagnosis of thoracic aortic rupture on plain film. *J. Emerg. Med.,* **1,** 21–28.

Feliciano D.V., Bitondo C.G., Mattox K.L. et al. (1984) The missed injury: sins in trauma care. *J. Trauma,* **24,** 657.

Feliciano D.V., Mattox K.L., Cruse P.A. et al. (1987) Delayed diagnosis of injuries to the diaphragm. *J. Trauma,* **27,** 821.

Harris R.D. and Harris J.H. (1988) The prevalence and significance of missed scapular fractures in blunt chest trauma. *Am. J. Radiol.,* **151,** 747–50.

Keen G. (1984) *Chest Injuries* 2nd edn, Bristol, Wright.

Weigelt J.A., Aurbakken C.M., Meier D.E. et al. (1982) Management of asymptomatic patients following stab wounds of the chest. *J. Trauma,* **22,** 291–4.

10   Abdominal injuries

The diagnosis of an intra-abdominal injury may be very easy in a shocked patient with evidence of abdominal wall trauma and with a rigid abdomen, but in many cases the signs are not nearly so straightforward at the time the patient is first seen, and missed or delayed diagnosis of abdominal injuries is one of the major causes of preventable trauma deaths (Anderson et al., 1988).

In a retrospective study of 20 patients with a ruptured spleen, the diagnosis was delayed for more than 12 hours in no fewer than 8, and 2 of these patients had been discharged home (McLauchlan et al., 1988). This study demonstrates the difficulty in diagnosing this injury as, at the time the patients were first seen, only 11 had left upper quadrant tenderness and in some of these patients this was attributed to the adjacent rib fractures. Only 7 had abdominal rigidity or guarding and other signs, such as pallor, hypotension and tachycardia, were even rarer. In 3 patients the diagnosis was made more difficult by a raised blood alcohol level.

Abdominal injuries are even more difficult to diagnose in the patient who has injuries elsewhere (Chapter 22). Other abdominal injuries may be equally difficult to diagnose.

Both bile (Michelassi and Ranson, 1985) and small bowel contents in the peritoneum may cause little inflammation initially, and injuries to retroperitoneal organs, e.g. duodenum and pancreas, are also difficult to diagnose.

If an intra-abdominal injury is diagnosed clinically, the patient will have a laparotomy immediately without further investigations, but other patients need further investigation. This investigation may be just to observe vital signs and to repeat the clinical examination of the abdomen at intervals, but more probably should be peritoneal lavage, ultrasound or CT. Laparoscopy may also be used and other investigations, e.g. contrast studies or isotope scans, may be done for specific injuries. Which investigation is used will depend on local facilities and experience, but each has its advantages and disadvantages and will also produce false positives and false negatives. Peritoneal lavage, for example, is very sensitive, but there may be false positives associated with trauma due to catheter placement, abdominal wall haematoma and extraperitoneal haematoma. False negatives may occur with extraperitoneal injuries, diaphragmatic hernia and if there are many adhesions. Complications may also occur (Soderstrom, Du Priest and Cowley, 1980). CT may not be reliable for hollow viscus and pancreatic injuries and its interpretation depends on experience (Peitzman et al., 1986). False positives also occur (Savitt, 1987).

The definitive investigation for abdominal injuries is a laparotomy which should be performed if, following investigations, an intra-abdominal injury has not been excluded. However, injuries may be missed even at laparotomy (Michelassi and Ranson, 1985; Scalea et al., 1988).

Haematuria or suspected urinary tract injury should be investigated with an intravenous urogram and/or a cystogram but a small percentage of ruptured bladders may fail to be demonstrated by these investigations (Sandler et al., 1986).

The standard management of penetrating abdominal injuries is a wound exploration and a full laparotomy in all patients in whom the peritoneum is breached but doing this results in a percentage of unnecessary laparotomies with their accompanying morbidity. A selective approach to the management of these injuries has, therefore, been recommended with the decision to operate depending on the results of clinical findings and/or peritoneal lavage. Results from published series have supported this selective approach, but injuries may still be missed, as with blunt injuries, including injuries missed at surgery (Feliciano et al., 1984, 1987). Penetrating abdominal injuries may also involve the chest and penetrating chest injuries may also involve the diaphragm, and so intra-abdominal injuries should be looked for in all penetrating chest injuries below the fourth intercostal space. Failure to do this will cause injuries to be missed (Feliciano et al., 1987).

Traumatic hernia is an uncommon condition which may be misdiagnosed as a haematoma (Guly, 1986). Failure to recognize it may lead to it being incised (Everett, 1973; Dubois and Freeman, 1981).

Practical points

- Abdominal pain following injury should be assumed to be due to an intra-abdominal injury until proved otherwise either by repeated examinations or preferably by ultrasound, CT or peritoneal lavage.
- Abdominal wall rigidity should not be attributed to rib fractures until intra-abdominal injury has been excluded by one of the investigations above.
- All investigations have false negatives, and so treat the patient, not the investigation. If there is any doubt as to whether there is an intra-abdominal injury, the patient must have a laparotomy.

REFERENCES

Anderson I.D., Woodford M., de Dombal F.T. et al. (1988) Retrospective study of 1,000 deaths from injury in England and Wales. *Br. Med. J.*, **296**, 1305–8.

Dubois P.M. and Freeman J.B. (1981) Traumatic abdominal wall hernia. *J. Trauma*, **21**, 72–74.

Everett W.G. (1973) Traumatic lumbar hernia. *Injury*, **4**, 354–6.

Feliciano D.V., Bitondo C.G., Mattox K.L et al. (1984) The missed injury: sins in trauma care. *J. Trauma*, **24**, 657.

Feliciano D.V., Mattox K.L., Cruse P.A., et al. (1987) Delayed diagnosis of injuries to the diaphragm. *J. Trauma*, **27**, 821.

Guly H.R. (1986) Beware the 'haematoma'. *Br. J. Acc. Emerg. Med.*, **1** (June), 16.

McLauchlan C.A.J., Maheson M., Sloan J.P. et al. (1988) Toward an earlier diagnosis of splenic injury. *Arch. Emerg. Med.*, **5**, 34–7.

Michelassi F. and Ranson J.H.C. (1985) Bile duct disruption by blunt trauma. *J. Trauma*, **25**, 454–7.

Peitzman A.B., Makaroun M.C., Slasky B.S. et al. (1986) Prospective study of computerised tomography in initial management of blunt abdominal trauma. *J. Trauma*, **26**, 585–92.

Sandler C.M., Hall J.T., Rodriguez M.B. et al. (1986) Bladder injury in blunt pelvic trauma. *Radiology,* **158,** 633–8.

Savitt R.M. (1987) Simulated splenic rupture on computerised tomography. *Br. J. Radiol.,* **60,** 713–4.

Scalea T.M., Phillips T.F., Goldstein A.S. et al (1988) Injuries missed at operation: nemesis of a trauma surgeon. *J. Trauma,* **28,** 962–7.

Soderstrom C.A., Du Priest R.W. and Cowley R.A. (1980) Pitfalls of peritoneal lavage in blunt abdominal trauma. *Surg. Gynecol. Obstet.,* **151,** 513–518.

11 Shoulder injuries

ANTERIOR DISLOCATION OF THE SHOULDER

This is a common injury which is usually easily recognized clinically and radiologically, but it can be missed (Schultz, Jacobs and Patterson, 1969; Rowe and Zarins, 1982). Missing a dislocation is more common in the elderly, in those unable to give a history of injury for whatever reason, and in the obese, in whom the typical deformity may be impossible to see or to palpate.

Nerve injuries in association with an anterior dislocation are uncommon, but will be missed unless specifically looked for.

POSTERIOR DISLOCATION OF THE SHOULDER

This is a rarer injury but unfortunately is more commonly missed (Schultz, Jacobs and Patterson, 1969; Rowe and Zarins, 1982; Hawkins et al., 1987) for a number of reasons.

Firstly, many posterior dislocations occur, not following direct injury, but following muscle spasm due to epileptic fits, electric shocks or (previously) unmodified ECT. To the knowledgeable, shoulder pain following one of these conditions instantly suggests the diagnosis, but the inexperienced may not appreciate that muscle spasm itself can cause such an injury.

Secondly, there is no obvious clinical deformity (although it is said that, if the shoulder is looked at from above, one can see an obvious bulge — I have never been convinced). However, in these patients, the arm is held in fixed internal rotation and cannot be got into a neutral position. This is a useful clinical sign to appreciate.

Lastly, these injuries are difficult to demonstrate on X-ray. An AP X-ray will usually show the 'lightbulb-on-end' appearance of a humeral head held in internal rotation (Figure 11.1a) (but this is not specific) and there may be incongruity between the head of the humerus and the glenoid, but many AP X-rays appear normal. The dislocation is easily shown on an axial shoulder X-ray (Figure 11.1b) but, following an injury, the patient is probably in severe pain and may be unwilling to abduct the arm enough to get the X-ray, and radiographers do not like to inflict the discomfort that may be required to get good X-rays. Alternative X-rays may then be done, but a lateral X-ray of the shoulder is usually uninterpretable and the trans-scapular lateral may also be difficult to interpret. If missed initially, these injuries may go unrecognized for months and years

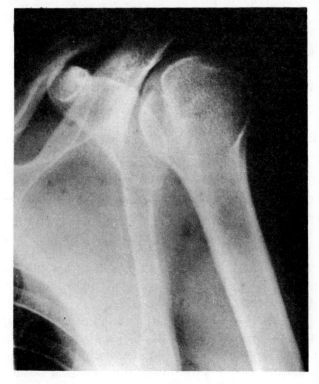

Figure 11.1a

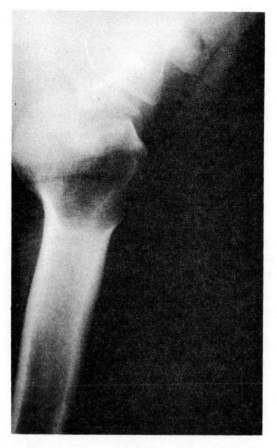

Figure 11.1b

Figure 11.1 Posterior dislocation of the shoulder. a, The AP X-ray looks normal except for the 'lightbulb-on-end' appearance of the humeral head showing that the humerus is internally rotated. b, An axial X-ray reveals the dislocation.

(33 years in the case of one patient [Rowe and Zarins, 1982]), and may be treated as a frozen shoulder with injections, manipulations and physiotherapy (Rowe and Zarins).

If a patient has the uncommon combination of posterior dislocation of the shoulder associated with a fractured shaft of humerus, the dislocation is even more likely to be missed (Barquet et al., 1985).

Missed bilateral shoulder dislocations are discussed in Chapter 22.

LONGSTANDING DISLOCATIONS

As some dislocated shoulders may be missed, and because some patients may not seek medical help following an injury, if such a patient re-injures the shoulder, the longstanding dislocation may be misdiagnosed as an acute injury (Guly, 1983), especially in the elderly or confused. If one is suspicious of an old injury, a surprisingly good range of movement may convince one that this is not a new injury, but usually one is reluctant to move what one imagines to be a recently dislocated shoulder. It is only when standard manoeuvres fail to reduce the dislocation that the true diagnosis becomes apparent.

The correct diagnosis of many other shoulder injuries depends on an accurate localization of the site of the injury, as not all injuries will be shown on a standard AP shoulder X-ray and they may require special views to be requested.

ACROMIOCLAVICULAR JOINT INJURIES

Subluxation and dislocation of the acromioclavicular joint may not be visible on an AP shoulder X-ray, especially if the patient is supine or has the arm supported in a sling, which will hold the dislocation reduced. To demonstrate this injury may require acromioclavicular views with the patient erect, possibly holding a weight in each hand, and comparison with the uninjured side.

A longstanding acromioclavicular dislocation may present as an acute injury.

STERNOCLAVICULAR JOINT INJURIES

These are best diagnosed clinically as, while there are various X-rays to demonstrate the sternoclavicular joint, none is ideal, and occasionally CT scanning is necessary to show the area. All dislocations of this joint are uncommon and posterior dislocations are rare, though they may be serious if the clavicle causes pressure on the trachea or neck vessels. Posterior dislocations are also easily missed (Worrell and Fernandez, 1986) but the clinical clue is pain in the base of the neck, made worse by shoulder movements.

SCAPULAR FRACTURES

Scapular fractures are usually the result of significant trauma and so are often associated with other injuries, when the scapular injury may be overlooked (Harris and Harris, 1988). In addition to an AP shoulder X-ray, a trans-scapular lateral and possibly an oblique X-ray must be done.

CORACOID FRACTURES

These are rare injuries, which may not be visible on standard X-rays, and require an axial X-ray. This may not be obtained for the reasons mentioned before, and the injury may be missed (De Rosa and Kettelkamp, 1977).

FALSE POSITIVE DIAGNOSES

The epiphysis at the upper end of the humerus is wedge-shaped and so on an AP X-ray two epiphyseal lines may be seen. The inexperienced casualty officer may confuse the more distal line for a fracture.

The ossification centre of the acromion may cause some confusion, as may an accessory bone at this site — the os acromionale.

The patient with a painful shoulder may sit slumped forward, with the scapula moved forward on the chest wall, causing the head of the humerus to be prominent. This may be felt clinically to be an anterior dislocation, but the X-rays will be normal.

Practical points

- Beware the epileptic with a frozen shoulder – it may be a posterior dislocation.
- In any patient with a shoulder injury following an epileptic fit or an electric shock and any patient with a fixed internal rotation deformity following an injury of whatever cause, you must get an axial X-ray to exclude a posterior dislocation.

  If you ask for this view, you must be prepared to assist the radiographer to get the arm into the position needed to take the X-ray. Give the patient some analgesia, entonox if necessary, and then very gentle, slow movement will usually do it. If you cannot get this view, ask for a trans-scapular lateral and seek help in its interpretation. Keep the patient under review and possibly get further X-rays later. Occasionally a trial of manipulation confirms the radiologically suspected but unproven diagnosis.

- Do not just ask for shoulder X-rays but localize the site of injury and specify what injury you suspect. The radiographer should then do appropriate views.

REFERENCES

Barquet A., Schimchak M., Carreros O. et al. (1985) Dislocation of the shoulder with fracture of the ipsilateral shaft of the humerus. *Injury,* **16,** 300–2.

Guly H.R. (1983) Longstanding dislocations presenting as acute injuries. *Br. J. Acc. Emerg. Med.,* (July), 13–14.

Harris R.D. and Harris J.H. (1988) The prevalence and significance of missed scapular fractures in blunt chest trauma. *Am J. Radiol.,* **151,** 747–50.

Hawkins R.J., Neer C.S., Pianta R.M. et al. (1987) Locked posterior dislocation of the shoulder. *J. Bone Jt Surg.,* **69A,** 9–18.

De Rosa P. and Kettelkamp D.B. (1977) Fracture of the coracoid process of the scapula. *J. Bone Jt Surg.,* **59A,** 696–7.

Rowe C.R. and Zarins B. (1982) Chronic unreduced dislocations of the shoulder. *J. Bone Jt Surg.,* **64A,** 494–505.

Schultz T.J., Jacobs B. and Patterson R.L. (1969) Unrecognised dislocations of the shoulder. *J. Trauma,* **9,** 1009–23.

Worrell J. and Fernandez G.N. (1986) Retrosternal dislocation of the sternoclavicular joint: an important injury easily missed. *Arch. Emerg. Med.,* **3,** 133–5.

12 Elbow and forearm injuries

ELBOW X-RAYS AND FRACTURES

The main diagnostic problem in the elbow is of demonstrating fractures on an X-ray. Standard elbow X-rays are an AP and a lateral, but these will not demonstrate all fractures and other views, including radial head and radial head capitellum (RHC) (Grundy et al., 1985) views can be done. Table 12.1 shows the result of a study (Hall-Graggs, Shorvon and Chapman, 1985) designed to show which views were best at diagnosing elbow fractures. Unfortunately, to diagnose every fracture, one needs every view.

Table 12.1 Demonstration of elbow fractures by different views (Hall-Craggs, Shorvon and Chapman, 1985)

31 patients with 32 elbow fractures	radial head	26
	olecranon	3
	coronoid	1
	radial head and capitellum	1

View	Fractures demonstated
AP and lateral	23
Radial head	26
RHC	16
AP and lateral RHC	29
Radial head and RHC	28

Radiological evidence of an elbow effusion following an injury is very important as a marker for fractures because a high proportion of patients with an effusion will have a fracture (82% in one series

[Smith and Lee, 1978]). If an effusion is present, one should look carefully for a fracture (two were missed in the above series) and, if necessary, do additional views (Figure 12.1).

Unfortunately not all fractures are seen on initial X-rays. Of the fractures in the above series (Smith and Lee) 39% were not detected on X-ray until follow-up X-rays were done. In another series of 35 patients with elbow effusions but no fractures seen on initial X-ray, repeat X-rays after 7–10 days showed 10 fractures of the radial head or neck (Morewood, 1987).

If it is essential that every elbow fracture must be diagnosed. A recommended protocol is (Hall-Craggs, Shorvon and Chapman, 1985):

All patients should have an AP and a lateral X-ray with radial head views if a fractured radial head is clinically suspected.

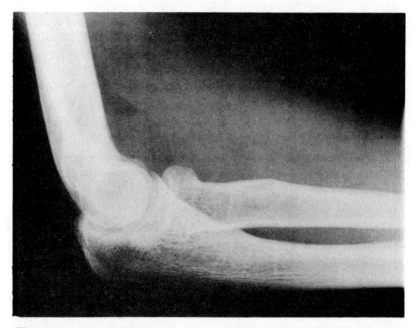

Figure 12.1 Fat pad sign. Note the soft-tissue lucencies in front of and behind the lower humerus indicating an effusion.

If these views show an effusion but no bony injury, a RHC view should be done.

If there is an effusion and none of these views show a fracture, they should be repeated after two weeks.

While this protocol will diagnose all fractures, it must be admitted that the chasing of fractures with repeat films after two weeks will not alter clinical management, as a radial head fracture or other fracture so small that it does not show on initial X-rays will be treated no differently from a patient with a traumatic effusion alone (Nutton, 1987; Welsh and McLauchlan, 1987; Wray, 1987). I give a compromise protocol below.

X-ray interpretation is even more difficult if standard views are not obtained. Sometimes this is because the patient is unable to move the elbow but, more often, it is because doctors try to diagnose elbow injuries on X-rays of the radius and ulna.

DISLOCATION OF THE RADIAL HEAD

Dislocation of the radial head is frequently missed both when it is an isolated injury (Wiley, Pegington and Horwich, 1974) or when it is part of a Monteggia fracture dislocation (9% [Letts, Locht and Weins, 1985] and 33% [Fowles, Sliman and Kassab, 1983] were missed in two recent series). If an isolated dislocation is missed and then diagnosed later, it may be assumed to be a congenital dislocation. The mistake can also be made the other way round, with a congenital dislocation of the radial head first being diagnosed when a child's elbow is X-rayed following an injury, and this congenital dislocation being diagnosed as a recent injury. However, the radial head which has never articulated with the capitellum is usually convex in appearance whereas the normal radial head is concave. Dislocation of the radial head should not be missed if the articulation between the radial head and the capitellum is specifically looked at on every elbow X-ray (Figure 12.2).

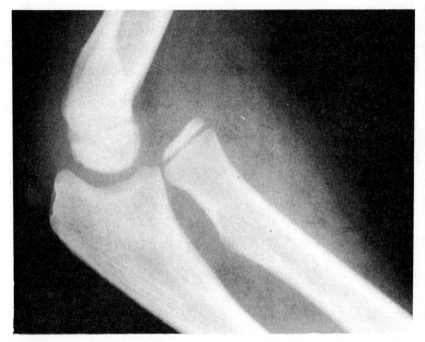

Figure 12.2 Dislocation of the radial head. The radial head is not articulating with the humerus.

PULLED ELBOW

The diagnosis of a pulled elbow in toddlers is usually easily made without recourse to X-rays by a classical history of a longitudinal pulling injury and physical examination showing full passive movements except for a block to supination, and the diagnosis is confirmed by the rapid response to manipulation. In the past it was poorly recognized and in 1954 7 cases were described, of which 2 had initially been diagnosed as brachial plexus injuries (Green and Gay, 1954). The condition has been better recognized since a larger series was described in a journal with more general readership (Illingworth, 1975) but many casualty officers have still never heard of it until after they start work in A & E. The condition is still occasionally thought initially to be a brachial plexus injury (personal knowledge) though the doctor is usually corrected by the nursing staff! It is still frequently over-investigated with unnecessary X-rays.

Recurrent episodes of pulled elbow may cause diagnostic difficulties if the history is not obtainable, and may present as 'recurrent paralysis of the arm' (Illingworth, 1975).

FRACTURES OF THE LATERAL CONDYLE OF THE ELBOW

These are important injuries, involving the articular surface of the elbow joint. Because, in children, much of the lateral condyle is cartilaginous and so not visible on X-ray, it is very easy to overlook them or to dismiss a minor radiological abnormality as being a minor fracture, whereas it may be a very serious injury.

TENNIS ELBOW

This is usually a chronic condition, and these are not considered in this book, but some cases may follow a direct blow to the lateral side of the elbow. These patients may present several weeks later with continuing pain, and are often diagnosed as 'elbow injury — X-ray NAD' which is true but unhelpful, as the treatable condition has been overlooked.

CLOSED AVULSIONS OF THE BICEPS AND TRICEPS TENDONS AT THE ELBOW

These injuries are rare and so may be overlooked. If doctors are aware that they can occur and know how to examine for them, they should not be missed (Figure 12.3).

FOREARM INJURIES

Isolated fractures of the midshaft of the radius or ulna do occur, but

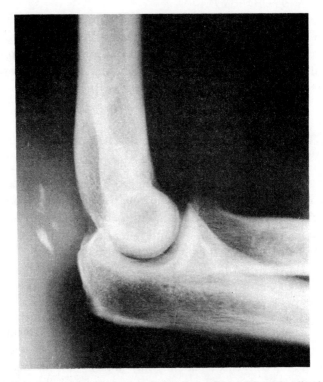

Figure 12.3 Not a chip fracture. Avulsion fractures should not be dismissed as chip fractures without first answering the question 'What has been avulsed?' In this case it was the triceps tendon.

they cannot displace to any degree without either the other bone fracturing or without a dislocation of the superior or inferior radio-ulnar joint. Mention has already been made about missing the radial head dislocation in Monteggia fractures (fractured shaft of the ulna with dislocation of the proximal radio-ulnar joint) but Galeazzi fractures (fracture of the radius with dislocation of the distal radio-ulnar joint) are also commonly misdiagnosed (Mikic, 1975).

FALSE POSITIVES

A major problem with diagnosing elbow injuries in children is the epiphyses, their appearances at different ages and the normal variation of epiphyses which may occur, such as fragmentation. When X-raying the elbow in children, the normal side should be X-rayed for comparison, either as a routine or certainly whenever there is any difficulty in interpreting the X-ray.

Congenital dislocation of the radial head presenting as an acute injury has been mentioned above.

Practical points

● When looking for elbow injuries, always request elbow X-rays and not forearm X-rays.
● Always ensure that you have a true lateral X-ray of the elbow.
● Learn to recognize the radiological appearance of an elbow effusion – the 'fat pad' sign.
● In children, X-ray the normal elbow for comparison.
● Always look at the articulation between the radius and the capitellum to exclude a dislocation.
● In patients with forearm fractures, ensure that you obtain X-rays of both elbow and wrist.
● What X-rays to order:
   Routine X-rays should be an AP and a lateral, with radial head X-rays if clinically indicated, and an AP and lateral X-ray of the other elbow in children. If the X-ray shows an effusion but no fracture, request RHC views.

If there is still no fracture seen, the patient will be given a sling for comfort and followed up in a clinic. Assuming in a clinic it is confirmed that the casualty officer has not missed a fracture, the patient should start to mobilize the arm, and the elbow can be X-rayed only if there are still significant symptoms at 2 weeks.

REFERENCES

Fowles J.V., Sliman N. and Kassab M.T. (1983) The Monteggia lesion in children. *J. Bone Jt Surg.*, **65A**, 1276–83.
Green J.T. and Gay F.H. (1954) Traumatic sublaxation of the radial head in young children. *J. Bone Jt Surg.*, **36A**, 655–62.

Grundy A., Murphy G., Barker A. et al. (1985) The value of the radial head – capitellum view in radial head trauma. *Br. J. Radiol.*, **58,** 965–7.

Hall-Craggs M.A., Shorvon P.J. and Chapman M. (1985) Assessment of the radial head – capitellum view and the dorsal fat pad sign in acute elbow trauma. *Am. J. Radiol.*, **145,** 607–9.

Illingworth C.M. (1975) Pulled elbow — a study of 100 patients. *Br. Med. J.*, **2,** 672–4.

Letts M., Locht R. and Weins J. (1985) Monteggia fracture dislocations in children. *J. Bone Jt Surg.*, **67B,** 724–7.

Mikic Z.D.J. (1975) Galeazzi fracture-dislocations. *J. Bone Jt Surg.*, **57A,** 1071–80.

Morewood D.J.W. (1987) Incidence of unsuspected fractures in traumatic effusions of the elbow joint. *Br. Med. J.*, **295,** 109–10.

Nutton R.W. (1987) Incidence of unsuspected fractures in effusions of the elbow. *Br. Med. J.*, **295,** 329.

Smith D.N. and Lee J.R. (1978) The radiological diagnosis of post-traumatic effusion of the elbow joint and its clinical significance: the 'displaced fat pad' sign. *Injury*, **10,** 115–9.

Welsh K.R. and McLauchlan C.A.J. (1987) Incidence of unsuspected fractures in traumatic effusions of the elbow. *Br. Med. J.*, **295,** 329–30.

Wiley J., Pegington J. and Horwich J.P. (1974) Traumatic dislocation of the radius at the elbow. *J. Bone Jt Surg.*, **56B,** 501–7.

Wray C. (1987) Incidence of unsuspected fractures in traumatic effusions of the elbow. *Br. Med. J.*, **295,** 329.

13 Wrist injuries

FRACTURES OF THE SCAPHOID

Scaphoid fractures are among the more common fractures presenting to A & E departments, and may be complicated by non-union, especially if untreated. This may cause later degenerative disease at the wrist. It is therefore important that they are correctly diagnosed but unfortunately they may be difficult to demonstrate on X-rays and are commonly missed. There are three main reasons why this happens.

Firstly, many scaphoid fractures may not be demonstrated on AP and lateral wrist X-rays. Failure to detect specific signs of scaphoid injury (especially anatomical snuff box tenderness and loss of wrist extension) will lead to wrist X-rays being requested rather than the 'scaphoid views' which are more likely to show the fracture.

Secondly, even if the fracture is visible on X-ray, it is one of the most commonly missed fractures (Wardrope and Chennells, 1985) (3% of fractures were missed in this way in one series [Leslie and Dickson, 1981]).

Lastly, about 2% of scaphoid fractures may not be visible on the original X-ray (Leslie and Dickson, 1981; Thomas, 1981; Young et al., 1988) and will only be seen on further films taken after an interval of 10–21 days. It has been suggested that those fractures which are not visible on initial X-rays will unite in any circumstances (Thomas, 1981) but, while this may be so for most patients, experience with individual patients suggests that it is not invariably true. Therefore all patients with clinical evidence of a fracture must be followed up in order that all fractures are diagnosed. This follow-up is usually to re-X-ray the patient following a period of immobilization. However, radio-isotope bone scans may be useful in that a negative scan excludes a fracture, thus allowing the soft-tissue injury to be treated earlier and avoiding unnecessary immobilization and further X-rays. In children, a much higher proportion of scaphoid fractures may not be visible on initial X-rays. Nafie (1987) found that initial X-rays were normal in 57% of waist fractures and 9% of distal pole fractures in children.

Some patients with a clinical diagnosis of fractured scaphoid may have other fractures (e.g. radial styloid and triquetrum) visible on the initial X-ray which may be missed (Duncan and Thurston, 1985; Da Cruz et al., 1988) or other fractures on repeat X-rays taken at three weeks (Da Cruz et al., 1988; Young et al., 1988). Other patients diagnosed by casualty officers to have clinical scaphoid fractures have specific soft-tissue diagnoses, such as tenosynovitis and traumatic ganglion (Da Cruz et al., 1988).

DISLOCATION OF THE LUNATE AND PERILUNAR DISLOCATION

Dislocations of the lunate and perilunar dislocations are uncommon injuries, with A & E departments seeing very few cases in a year. While they should easily be diagnosed on a lateral wrist X-ray if looked for, the appearances on an AP X-ray are subtle and this, combined with their rarity, leads to these injuries being missed very frequently (Figure 13.1).

Unfortunately, delayed treatment leads to a worse prognosis (Rawlings, 1981). In two series, only 54% (Rawlings, 1981) and 66% (Panting et al., 1984) were diagnosed within 24 hours, the delay in diagnosis in the rest ranging from one day to 18 months. Reasons for the delayed diagnosis were failure to recognize the injury on an X-ray and also when it occurred in patients with multiple injuries. Dislocation of the lunate may be associated with other injuries in the wrist or hand, and this leads to it being missed while a more obvious injury is diagnosed and treated (Juhl and Saether, 1987).

Trans-scapho-perilunar dislocation is another uncommon injury which may be missed, though usually the X-ray is recognized as being abnormal, even if the casualty officer fails to recognize what the abnormality is.

FRACTURE OF THE HOOK OF THE HAMATE

Fractures of the hook of the hamate are even rarer than lunate dislocations and are even more commonly missed because they are not seen on standard X-rays but require a carpal tunnel view of the wrist to show them. They may be caused by a fall on the outstretched hand or, more usually, by a localized force over the area

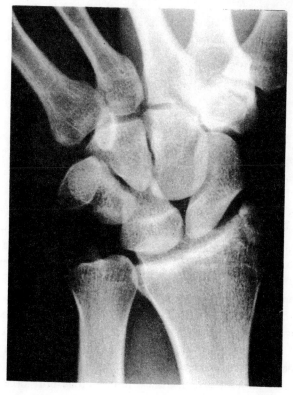

Figure 13.1a

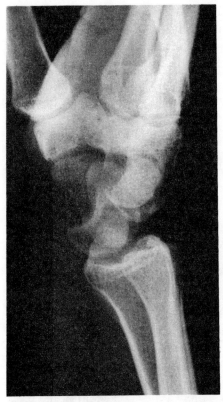

Figure 13.1 Dislocation of the lunate. a, the AP X-ray shows a fractured radial styloid (which was diagnosed) but otherwise it could be passed as normal (and was). However, note the triangular appearance of the lunate. b, The lateral X-ray demonstrates the dislocation.

Figure 13.1b

as occurs when a golfer hits the ground with his club. The symptoms and signs are pain in the ulna side of the hand, made worse on gripping, with point tenderness over the hook of the hamate in the hypothenar eminence (Carter, Eaton and Littler, 1977). In one series of 9 cases, none was correctly diagnosed initially (Carter, Eaton and Littler) and, in another series of 20 cases, only 3 had been correctly diagnosed initially (Stark et al., 1977). The rest had had symptoms for up to four years and had frequently been misdiagnosed as sprained wrist or tendinitis, and had been injected with steroids before the diagnosis was made and the condition treated by excision of the fractured hook. Rarely these injuries may only be diagnosed on a CT scan (Mizuseki, 1986).

GREENSTICK FRACTURE OF THE LOWER RADIUS

The minor greenstick or 'buckle' fracture of the distal end of the radius is a common injury, which is frequently not recognized (Wardrope and Chennells, 1985), particularly by new casualty officers who think that, to diagnose a fracture, they need to see a cortical break or a line across a bone, and ignore the slight angulation.

This is a minor fracture which causes little or no harm if untreated but, when missed for this reason, it indicates inadequate teaching on the nature of fractures.

CHIP FRACTURE FROM THE DORSUM OF THE TRIQUETRUM

This is another common but minor injury, usually only seen on the lateral wrist X-ray, but which is frequently missed or not recognized as a fracture.

SMITH'S FRACTURE

The deformity of a Smith's fracture may be diagnosable clinically but frequently there is much swelling over the dorsum of the wrist, obscuring the deformity and giving the clinical appearance of a Colles fracture. The X-ray will confirm the anterior angulation and displacement of a Smith's fracture, but occasionally the X-ray is inadequately looked at and the deformity wrongly diagnosed, so it is manipulated as a Colles fracture.

COLLES FRACTURE AND ASSOCIATED INJURIES

Colles fractures are common and are usually easily diagnosed, but what is not always recognized is that a patient with a Colles fracture may also have other injuries (Smith et al., 1988). In a series of 565 patients with Colles fractures, 12 (2.1%) had associated injuries not recognized at presentation (Cooney, Dobyns and Linscheid, 1980). These comprised 4 scaphoid fractures, 2 radial head fractures, 1 Bennett's fracture and 5 intercarpal ligament injuries.

Scaphoid fractures, too, may be associated with other injuries (Funk and Wood, 1988).

FALSE POSITIVES

As described above, scaphoid fractures are easily missed, and sometimes the patient may not have sought medical help. Many a scaphoid fracture is first diagnosed years later, when the wrist is X-rayed following another injury. However, the radiological signs of established non-union and, often, secondary degenerative changes, should not cause this to be misdiagnosed as a recent injury.

The numerous accessory bones which may occur at the wrist and the occasional old chip fracture may be misdiagnosed as an acute injury, but the fact that these are well rounded, with a cortex all round, usually proves that they are of long standing.

Fractured scaphoids are greatly over-diagnosed. Many patients with pain on the radial side of the wrist are diagnosed as having a 'clinical scaphoid fracture', even when there is no history of trauma, or the mechanism of injury is such that it would not cause a scaphoid fracture. The two conditions most commonly misdiagnosed in this way are de Quervain's syndrome and osteoarthritis of the first carpometacarpal joint. Apart from sloppy thinking about the mechanism of injury, the reason for these misdiagnoses is failure to localize the pain exactly.

Practical points

● If you suspect a scaphoid injury, ask for scaphoid X-rays not wrist X-rays.
● If there is anatomical snuff box tenderness but X-rays are normal, arrange for the patient to be reviewed in 10–14 days for re-X-ray if symptoms persist (unless your hospital investigates such patients with bone scans)

If the patient has other signs of scaphoid fracture, such as swelling and loss of wrist extension, treat him as for a fracture in a scaphoid plaster and arrange for his review.

● Every time you look at a lateral wrist X-ray, ask yourself 'Is this lunate dislocated?' even if the patient has other injuries.

● Whenever you see a lateral X-ray of a Colles fracture, check which way the deformity is (N.B. the first metacarpal is anterior).

● Even if the patient has an obvious fracture, still go round every bone on the X-ray with a finger, as he may have other injuries as well.

REFERENCES

Carter P.R., Eaton R.G. and Littler J.W. (1977) Ununited fracture of the hook of the hamate. *J. Bone Jt Surg.,* **59A,** 583–8.

Cooney W.P., Dobyns J.H. and Linscheid R.L. (1980) Complications of Colles fracture. *J. Bone Jt Surg.,* **62A,** 613–9.

Da Cruz D.J., Taylor R.H., Savage B. et al. (1988) Ultrasound assessment of the fractured scaphoid. *Arch. Emerg. Med.,* **5,** 97–100.

Duncan D.S. and Thurston A.J. (1985) Clinical fracture of the carpal scaphoid — an illusionary diagnosis. *J. Hand Surg.,* **10B,** 375–6.

Funk D.A. and Wood M.B. (1988) Concurrent fractures of the ipsilateral scaphoid and radial head. *J. Bone Jt Surg.,* **70A,** 134–6.

Juhl M. and Saether J. (1987) Simultaneous dislocation of the interphalangeal joint of the thumb and the carpal lunate. *J. Trauma,* **27,** 581–2.

Leslie I.J. and Dickson R.A. (1981) The fractured scaphoid. Natural history and factors influencing outcome. *J. Bone Jt Surg.,* **63B,** 225–30.

Mizuseki T., Ikuta Y., Murakami T. et al. (1986) Lateral approach to the hook of the hamate for its fracture. *J. Hand Surg.,* **11B,** 109–11.

Nafie S.A.A. (1987) Fractures of the carpal bones in children. *Injury,* **18,** 117–9.

Panting A.L., Lamb D.W., Noble J. et al. (1984) Dislocations of the lunate with and without fracture of the scaphoid. *J. Bone Jt Surg.,* **66B,** 391–5.

Rawlings I.D. (1981) The management of dislocations of the carpal lunate. *Injury,* **12,** 319–30.

Smith J.T., Keeve J.P., Bertin K.C. et al. (1988) Simultaneous fractures of the distal radius and scaphoid. *J. Trauma,* **28,** 676–9.

Stark H.H., Jobe F.W., Boyes J.H. et al. (1977) Fracture of the hook of the hamate in athletes. *J. Bone Jt Surg.,* **59A,** 575–82.

Thomas T.L. (1981) Some aspects of the fractured scaphoid. *J. R. Soc. Med.,* **74,** 800–3.

Wardrope J. and Chennells P.M. (1985) Should all casualty radiographs be reviewed? *Br. Med. J.*, **290**, 1638–40.

Young M.R.A., Lowry J.H., McLeod N.W. et al. (1988) Clinical carpal scaphoid injuries. *Br. Med. J.*, **296**, 825–6.

14　Hand injuries

Although the hand is a common site for missed injuries, most of these are tendon and nerve injuries which are discussed in Chapter 18. Some joint injuries are regularly missed, and these are described below. Hand injuries are important and, sometimes, although an injury has been correctly diagnosed, its significance and the need for it to be treated may not be recognized (Finlayson et al., 1986).

CARPOMETACARPAL (CMC) DISLOCATION

Dislocation of the first CMC joint is not an uncommon injury, but it may be missed (Johnson, Jones and Hoddincott, 1987). Dislocation of the other CMC joints are uncommon injuries but, when they do occur, they usually affect the fifth or the fourth and fifth joints, and they are commonly missed (Henderson and Arafa, 1987). In a recent series of 21 cases, 15 were missed in A & E and 5 of these were also missed by orthopaedic consultants or senior registrars, the diagnosis being delayed for up to four months (Editorial, 1987). The clinical features are of a bony lump at the base of the metacarpal (but this may initially be masked by soft-tissue swelling) and slight ulna deviation of the little finger. In many hospitals 'routine' hand X-rays consist of an AP and an oblique X-ray, and in these views the signs of a CMC dislocation are subtle. A lateral X-ray of the hand is needed to diagnose the injury (Figure 14.1).

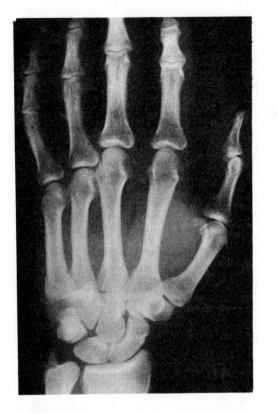 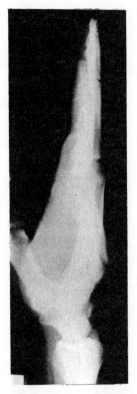

Figure 14.1a   **Figure 14.1b**

Figure 14.1 Dislocation of the 5th carpometacarpal joint. a, The AP X-ray was accepted as normal but it is not — compare it with Fig. 14.2a. b, The dislocation is seen on the lateral X-ray.

FRACTURES AROUND AND FRACTURE DISLOCATIONS OF THE PROXIMAL INTERPHALANGEAL (PIP) JOINT

These are easily missed on a hand X-ray, but will not be missed if the finger is X-rayed (Figure 14.2). This has been discussed in Chapter 3.

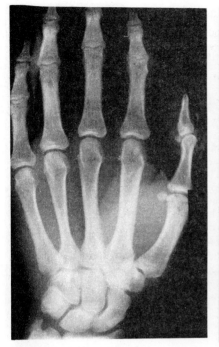
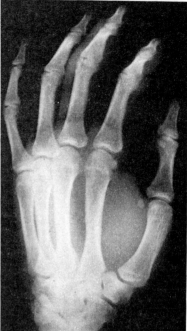

Figure 14.2a   **Figure 14.2b**

DISLOCATIONS OF THE PROXIMAL AND DISTAL INTERPHALANGEAL JOINTS

These are usually easily diagnosed clinically and easily reduced, and this is frequently done by the patient, who may not even come to hospital. However, what is suitable management on the rugby pitch is not suitable in hospital, and it is important that these injuries are documented and a post-reduction X-ray obtained. This is partly to exclude associated fractures and also because it is not unknown for patients to dislocate both finger joints. If the PIP joint is just 'pulled straight' and the patient discharged, by the time the patient returns complaining of a stiff DIP joint, it may be impossible to do a closed reduction of the dislocation, and an open reduction will be necessary.

◀ Figure 14.2c

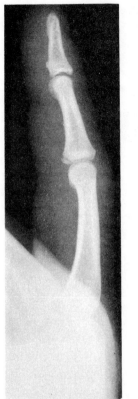

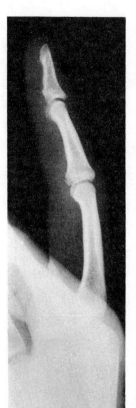

Figure 14.2 X-ray the injured part. The patient injured the index and middle fingers. a, b, Initially the hand was X-rayed which missed the injuries. c, d, X-rays of the fingers showed fractures of both PIP joints.

Figure 14.2d ▶

Isolated dislocations of the distal interphalangeal joint are easy to overlook clinically or to be diagnosed clinically as a fractured distal phalanx that does not need an X-ray.

FRACTURES AT THE BASE OF THE DISTAL PHALANX (DP)

Fractures at the base of the distal phalanx, especially minimally displaced epiphyseal fractures, will cause swelling, and the inflammatory response which occurs as part of the healing process may cause redness and warmth, and so these injuries may be misdiagnosed as paronychias (Guly, 1986) (and personal knowledge of other cases).

LIGAMENTOUS INJURIES

Ligament ruptures, especially of the ulna collateral ligament of the first MCP joint and the radial collateral ligaments of the PIP joints, are important injuries which may be amenable to surgical repair (especially the first MCP joint injury). These injuries will certainly be missed if joint stability is not tested (if necessary under local anaesthetic). On X-ray, important ligament avulsion fractures should be recognized for what they are, and not dismissed as 'chip fractures'.

LOCKED FINGER

A locked MCP joint (locked finger) in which a patient, either spontaneously or following a minor injury, is unable fully to extend the MCP joint either actively or passively, is an uncommon problem which is poorly described in textbooks and often not recognized even by more senior orthopaedic staff. It is usually thought clinically to be a dislocation of the MCP joint and then, when an X-ray shows no dislocation, it may be misdiagnosed as a trigger finger (Bruner, 1961; Fernandez, 1988).

FALSE POSITIVES

Various sesamoid bones may be visible on a hand X-ray. These are usually well rounded and corticated and do not usually confuse, but the sesamoid at the base of the distal phalanx of the thumb on the volar aspect is sometimes misdiagnosed as an avulsion fracture.

Nutrient arteries in the metacarpals are sometimes misdiagnosed as fractures.

Soft-tissue calcification of various causes, e.g. acute calcific periarthritis, may be misdiagnosed as a chip fracture (Carroll, Sirton and Garcia, 1955).

Practical points

- If clinically you suspect CMC dislocation either because of significant swelling on the dorsum of the hand in that area or because the standard hand X-rays are 'not right', you must get a lateral X-ray of the hand.
- Finger injuries are best shown (and may only be shown) on finger X-rays, not a hand X-ray. Similarly, for thumb injuries, ask for the thumb and not the hand to be X-rayed.
- Testing for stability is part of the routine examination of any joint. If there is swelling of the PIP joint or of the first MCP joint, always test for stability.

REFERENCES

Bruner J.M. (1961) Recurrent locking of the index finger due to internal derangement of the metacarpophalangeal joint. *J. Bone Jt Surg.*, **43A**, 450–2.

Carroll R.E., Sirton W. and Garcia A. (1955) Acute calcium deposits in the hand. *JAMA*, **157**, 422–6.

Editorial (1987) Slap on the wrist for another missed diagnosis. *Lancet*, **i**, 1772.

Fernandez G.N. (1988) Locking of a metacarpophalangeal joint caused by a haemangioma of the volar plate. *J. Hand Surg.*, **13B**, 323–4.

Finlayson B.J., Cross A.B., Shalley M.J. et al. (1986) The value of a next day hand injury review clinic. *J. Hand Surg.*, **11B**, 438–40.

Guly H.R. (1986) Fractures not X-rayed. *Arch. Emerg. Med.*, **3**, 159–62.

Henderson J.J. and Arafa M.A.M. (1987) Carpometacarpal dislocations: an easily missed diagnosis. *J. Bone Jt Surg.*, **69B**, 212–4.

Johnson S.R., Jones D.G. and Hoddincott H.C. (1987) Missed carpometacarpal dislocation of the thumb in motorcyclists. *Injury*, **18**, 415–6.

15 Hip and pelvic injuries

FRACTURED NECK OF FEMUR

Femoral neck fractures are very common in the elderly and are also commonly missed. In one series, 5.3% of patients had their fractures (mostly undisplaced) missed (Eastwood, 1987), with incorrect diagnoses being made of exacerbation of osteoarthritis of the hip, hemiparesis, rheumatoid arthritis and pain due to a previous injury. Factors involved in the missed diagnoses were confused patients, a lack of any history of trauma and also a history of frequent falls. In the same series, another 1.3% of patients had the diagnosis suspected, but it was difficult to confirm. This category of patients was also looked at by Fairclough and colleagues (1987), who examined 693 elderly patients with suspected hip fractures. Of these patients 43 had normal hip X-rays and these underwent an isotope bone scan, 13 of which were positive, and these patients were found to have fractures. Thus 13 out of 663 (2%) patients with fractured necks of femur had normal X-rays initially.

Others have also commented on the difficulty in diagnosing hip fractures in patients without any history of injury (Franklin, 1979) and in patients who already have chronic hip pain due to some other cause (Williams, Amin and Young, 1986).

The hip is examined with the patient lying down, and it is not uncommon to find a full range of hip movements. On this evidence, the doctor assumes that there is no need to X-ray the patient, without ever examining the patient's gait. It is also common to assume that, because the patient can walk, there is no fracture. Neither of these assumptions is true, and both will miss the initially undisplaced fracture which may displace later.

Some fractures may also be missed on X-ray especially if only an AP X-ray and no lateral is taken. Degenerative disease of the hip may make fractures difficult to see.

A fractured femoral neck may rarely occur in association with a fractured femoral shaft. In these cases, the femoral neck fracture is easily missed (Shaheen and Badr, 1987).

FRACTURES OF THE PUBIC RAMI

Fractures of the pubic rami, while much less important, are also common in the elderly and need to be looked for particularly in the patient who falls and has pain although there is no femoral neck fracture. They are commonly missed for the same reasons.

SLIPPED UPPER FEMORAL EPIPHYSIS

At the other end of the age range, slipped upper femoral epiphysis is also frequently missed initially (Brenkel, Prosser and Pearce, 1986), resulting in a worse prognosis. Some, but not all, give a history of trauma or an acute onset. A series of 300 slipped epiphyses (Wilson, Jacobs and Schecter, 1965) showed that many patients had had symptoms for six months before the diagnosis was made and that 26% had had false diagnoses. The most common was muscle strain, and others included Osgood–Schlatter's disease, flat feet and growing pains. One cause of the problem is that the pain is frequently felt in the thigh or the knee (Wilson, Jacobs and Schecter), which leads to the wrong part of the limb being examined and possibly X-rayed. Another problem is that, because there is a reluctance to expose the adolescent pelvis to radiation, if a child does complain of hip or knee pain, only an AP X-ray of the pelvis may be done. In the early stages this may be normal, and a lateral X-ray (or frog leg lateral) is required to show the slip.

DISLOCATION OF THE HIP

Traumatic posterior dislocation of the hip causes a typical deformity, with the hip being held flexed, adducted and internally rotated, and so should never be missed. However, this may happen if the patient has other significant lower limb injuries, which may divert attention from the hip or mask the deformity (Nixon, 1976). In particular, fractures of the shaft of the femur may be associated with dislocation of the hip and in these cases the dislocation may be overlooked (Helal and Skevis, 1967). The clinical signs of a dislocated hip in association with a femoral shaft fracture have been described (Helal and Skevis) but, if the basic radiological rules of X-raying the joint above and below any long bone fracture are kept, dislocations should be picked up and it should not be necessary to look for these signs.

On occasions the AP X-ray may look relatively normal but the dislocation will be shown on the lateral, though this may be difficult to obtain.

Many dislocated hips are associated with fractures of the acetabulum. Uncommonly they may be associated with fractures of the head of the femur and these important fractures may be misdiagnosed as being from the acetabulum (Lang-Stevenson and Getty, 1987).

Dislocations of the hip may be complicated by sciatic nerve palsy, and this should be looked for.

PELVIC FRACTURES

Fractures of the acetabulum and pelvis are usually easily seen on X-rays, but standard X-rays may not fully show the extent of the fracture and further investigations may be required, particularly if surgery is planned.

As well as fully demonstrating the fracture, CT scanning may also show additional pelvic fractures, especially of the sacrum and sacro-iliac joint, which were not seen on the standard X-rays (Dunn, Berry and Connally, 1983).

In patients with multiple injuries, pelvic fractures may not be diagnosed clinically but they are of great importance, not least because of the blood loss which may be associated with them. The pelvis should, therefore, be X-rayed routinely in all patients with multiple injuries.

Avulsion fractures from the pelvis are considered in Chapter 18.

FALSE POSITIVES

In children, the varying appearance of the triradiate cartilage may give the appearance of a fracture.

The os acetabuli, an accessary bone just above the acetabulum, may be confused with a chip fracture of the acetabulum.

Practical points

● Always X-ray the pelvis of any elderly patient who:
   (a) Falls and complains of pain anywhere between the waist and the knee.
   (b) Complains of hip pain or an exacerbation of chronic hip pain even in the absence of any history of injury.
   (c) Goes off his feet without any apparent reason.
● Always get a lateral X-ray of the hip, too.
● The patient who falls, injuring the hip, and who has a normal X-ray may still have a fracture. He may need admission anyway for rehabilitation, but if he continues to complain of hip pain, he should have a bone scan or repeat X-rays after an interval.
● If a child complains of pain in the knee, but the knee is normal to examination — examine the hip as well. If there is any possibility of a slipped upper femoral epiphysis, do AP and lateral (or frog leg lateral) hip X-rays.
● If a patient has a fractured femur, ensure you have an X-ray of the hip.
● X-ray the pelvis in all patients with multiple injuries.

REFERENCES

Brenkel I.J., Prosser A.J. and Pearce M. (1986) Slipped capital femoral epiphysis: continuing problem of late diagnosis. *Br. Med. J.,* **293,** 256–7.

Dunn E.L., Berry P.H. and Connally J.D. (1983) Computed tomography of the pelvis in patients with multiple injuries. *J. Trauma,* **23,** 378–83.

Eastwood H.D.H. (1987) Delayed diagnosis of femoral neck fracture in the elderly. *Age and Aging,* **16,** 378–82.

Fairclough J., Colhoun E., Johnston D. et al. (1987) Bone scanning for suspected hip fractures. *J. Bone Jt Surg.,* **69B,** 251–3.

Franklin P. (1979) A 'silent' fracture of the femoral neck. *Hospital Update,* Dec. p. 188.

Helal B. and Skevis X. (1967) Unrecognised dislocation of the hip in fractures of the femoral shaft. *J. Bone Jt Surg.,* **49B,** 293-300.

Lang-Stevenson A. and Getty C.J.M. (1987) The Pipkin fracture-dislocation of the hip. *Injury,* **18,** 264–9.

Nixon J.R. (1976) Late open reduction of traumatic dislocation of the hip. *J. Bone Jt Surg.,* **58B,** 41–3.

Shaheen M.A.E.K. and Badr A.A. (1987) Concomitant ipsilateral femoral shaft and femoral neck fractures. *J. R. Coll. Surg. Edinb.,* **32,** 223–7.

Williams P.L., Amin N.K. and Young A. (1986) Unsuspected fractures of the femoral neck in patients with chronic hip pain due to rheumatoid arthritis. *Br. Med. J.,* **292,** 1125–6.

Wilson P.D., Jacobs R. and Schecter L. (1965) Slipped capital femoral epiphysis. *J. Bone Jt Surg.,* **47A,** 1128–45.

16 Knee and leg injuries

LIGAMENTOUS AND MENISCAL INJURIES

Initial assessment of knee injuries depends on an accurate history, including details of any previous injuries, and a full examination. If this is not done, then injuries will be (and are) missed. However, these injuries may occur in combination as well as singly, and it may be difficult or impossible to make an accurate and complete diagnosis on clinical findings alone. This may also require an examination under anaesthetic, arthroscopy and possibly arthrography.

In one series of 100 patients who were fully investigated, the clinical diagnosis was correct in 72% and in another 10% it was correct but incomplete, and in 18% of patients the clinical diagnosis was incorrect (De Haven and Collins, 1975). In another series of 118 patients, a total of 174 ligamentous or meniscal injuries were found. Only 61·5% were diagnosed clinically and there were also 74 false positive diagnoses (Simonsen et al., 1984).

To provide a complete diagnosis of knee injuries is therefore costly and requires a general anaesthetic. Whether this is justified or necessary will depend on whether treatment and prognosis are likely to be altered as a result. There are clearly many variables involved, and this book is not the place to discuss the alternative treatments available and their benefits.

Orthopaedic surgeons need to draw up criteria (preferably based on facts rather than opinions) as to which patients will benefit from further investigations, and the aim in an A & E department should be to diagnose those soft tissue injuries that are diagnosable, and also to diagnose those patients who require further investigation.

Ligamentous injuries of the knee are often missed because stability is not tested.

DISLOCATION AND FRACTURES OF THE PATELLA

The occasional patient presents with a dislocated patella and this is an easy clinical diagnosis. However, more often the dislocated patella will have reduced spontaneously, and the diagnosis of this injury depends on obtaining the history that the patella moved laterally and then went back again. If this detailed history is not obtained, the diagnosis will be missed.

Dislocation of the patella may be associated with marginal or osteochondral fractures. The latter particularly need to be diagnosed as otherwise they form a loose body in the joint. Unfortunately they are frequently missed (De, 1983) if not looked for with a full set of patella X-rays. Some osteochondral fractures seen at surgery may not be visible on X-rays (Jensen and Roosen, 1985).

Many patella fractures may not be visible on standard knee X-rays. In one series of patella fractures, AP and lateral X-rays alone would have missed 14% which were only visible on oblique X-rays (Daffner and Tabas, 1987). Axial (skyline) X-rays of the patella are also useful.

EPIPHYSEAL FRACTURES OF THE LOWER FEMUR AND UPPER TIBIA

Some epiphyseal fractures, especially those of the lower femoral epiphysis, may be undisplaced initially and thus not show on initial X-rays (Rang, 1974; Bernard and Evans, 1986), but they may displace later. Examination of such knees for stability under anaesthetic (and possibly without anaesthetic) will cause movement at the fracture site, thereby mimicking a ligamentous injury (O'Brien, Warren and Gollehon, 1988). All children who seem to have a severe sprain of the knee or a ligamentous injury should have a stress X-ray.

OSTEOCHONDRAL FRACTURES OF THE LATERAL FEMORAL CONDYLE

These need open reduction and internal fixation in order to prevent loose body formation. Unfortunately they are frequently missed in both A & E and fracture clinics, despite being visible on standard knee X-rays (Matthewson and Dandy, 1978). If there is any doubt, an intercondylar (tunnel) X-ray should be done.

FLAKE FRACTURES

Flake fractures around the knee should not be dismissed as 'chip fractures' as they usually represent important ligamentous injuries (Fairclough and Johnson, 1988).

LACERATIONS INTO THE KNEE JOINT

Lacerations around the knee joint may involve the joint, and these compound joint injuries need to be treated with the same respect given to compound fractures. In all lacerations around the knee (or any other large joint), the joint should be X-rayed. Air in the joint (seen as an air/fluid level on a horizontal beam lateral X-ray) indicates that the wound enters the joint (Figure 16.2).

Injuries of the quadriceps tendon and patella ligament are discussed in Chapter 18.

SPIRAL FRACTURES OF THE TIBIA IN TODDLERS

These are common but are not serious, which is just as well as they are frequently overlooked. The child falls and will not weight bear. Tenderness is difficult to localize in the crying child, and there will be a full range of seemingly painless hip, knee and ankle movements. Initial X-rays are frequently normal. The initial diagnosis is thus a clinical one based on suspicion and experience rather than evidence, but further X-rays at two weeks (by which time the child is often better) will show either a fracture line or, more usually, just periosteal elevation.

FRACTURES OF THE FIBULA

Fractures of the upper and middle third of the fibula are usually relatively minor injuries, and the patient may continue his activities and present late. Because of this, the doctor may feel that an X-ray is not indicated and so the fracture is missed, though there is no specific treatment and no harm results.

FALSE POSITIVES

1. A bipartite patella may be misdiagnosed as a fracture but its appearance as a well-rounded bony fragment in the upper lateral quadrant of the patella is not at all like a fracture (Figure 16.1). Other rarer variants of patella ossification may also cause confusion. If in doubt, the other knee can be X-rayed, as this is often bilateral.
2. The fabella, a sesamoid bone in the tendon of the lateral head of the gastrocnemius, may be misdiagnosed as a loose body.
3. A minor knee injury may, by the following day, have a large effusion, but the history that the patient was able to finish the game of football will usually exclude a serious knee injury.
4. A longstanding ligamentous laxity may masquerade as a new injury.
5. A history of the knee 'giving way' usually suggests a mechanical cause, but quadriceps wasting (e.g. from a previous injury not fully rehabilitated) will cause the same problem.

PRACTICAL POINTS

● Knee injuries are difficult to diagnose. An accurate history, including past history, mechanism of injury and what happened after the injury, is essential, as is a full examination.

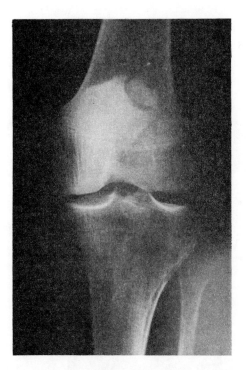

Figure 16.1 Normal variant
— bipartite patella. Note the
separate ossification centre in
the upper lateral part of the
patella. It is well rounded and
not like a fracture.

- Beware the patient with a severe knee injury but no effusion as this usually represents a major ligamentous injury. If the capsule has been torn, the expected haemarthrosis will be in the soft tissues around the knee.
- With all patella injuries, request patella X-rays as well as knee X-rays.
- If you suspect a loose body, request an intercondylar (tunnel) view.
- Always X-ray the knee if there is a deep laceration around it. Air in the knee joint proves that the laceration involves the joint.
- Ask advice about all children with severe knee injuries, as they may need stress X-rays to exclude an epiphyseal fracture.
- Following trauma, a liparthrosis (shown by a fluid level on a horizontal beam lateral X-ray or seen in the aspirate following knee aspiration) must indicate a fracture. If you cannot see it – look at the X-rays again.

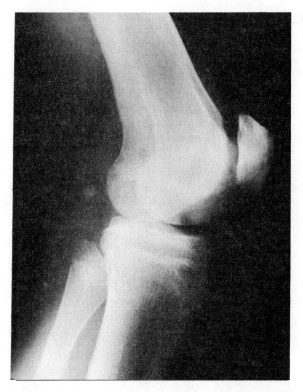

Figure 16.2 Air in the knee joint. The patient had a wound in the vicinity of the knee. An X-ray shows no bony injury but there is air in the joint indicating that the wound enters the joint. Note also the accessory bone (fabella) which can be misdiagnosed as a loose body in the joint.

REFERENCES

Bernard A.A. and Evans D.A. (1986) Missed lower femoral epiphyseal injury. *J. R. Coll. Surg. Edinb.*, **31,** 194–5.

De D. (1983) Osteochondral fracture of the patella. *Br. J. Acc. Emerg. Med.,* **1** July, p. 19.

Daffner R.H. and Tabas J.H. (1987) Trauma oblique radiographs of the knee. *J. Bone Jt Surg.,* **69A,** 568–72.

Fairclough J.A. and Johnson S.R. (1988) Ski injuries, the significance of flake fractures. *Injury,* **19,** 79–80.

De Haven K.E. and Collins H.R. (1975) Diagnosis of internal derangement of the knee. *J. Bone Jt Surg.,* **57A,** 802–10.

Jensen C.M. and Roosen J.M. (1985) Acute traumatic dislocations of the patella. *J. Trauma,* **25,** 160–2.

Mathewson M.H. and Dandy D.J. (1978) Osteochondral fractures of the lateral femoral condyle. *J. Bone Jt Surg.,* **60B,** 199–202.

O'Brien S., Warren R.F. and Gollehon D. (1988) Intra-articular fracture of the femur mimicking insufficiency of the posterior cruciate ligament. *J. Bone Jt Surg.,* **70A,** 461–2.

Rang M. (1974) *Children's Fractures,* 2nd edn, Philadelphia, Lippincott.

Simonsen O., Jensen J., Mouritsen P. et al. (1984) The accuracy of clinical examination of the knee joint. *Injury,* **16,** 96–100.

17   Ankle and foot injuries

INDICATIONS FOR X-RAY

Ankle injuries (especially inversion injuries) are very common and, unless every injured ankle is X-rayed which is impractical (especially in general practice) and probably inappropriate, decisions need to be made as to whom to X-ray in order to diagnose all (or at least all significant) fractures. If the wrong decision is made, injuries will be missed. Various doctors have investigated the clinical features which indicate the probability of a fracture, and these are summarized in Table 17.1.

Table 17.1 Clinical indicators of an ankle fracture

Age >60 (Garfield, 1960; Dunlop et al., 1986)

Age >40 (Vargish et al., 1983)

Bony tenderness (Brand et al., 1982; Vargish et al., 1983;
           Dunlop et al., 1986)

Inability to weight bear (Dunlop et al., 1986)

History of a direct blow to the ankle (Vargish et al., 1983)

Clinical indicators of the absence of a significant fracture

Absence of swelling (Garfield, 1960; de Lacey and Bradbrooke, 1979)

Tenderness over the anterior fibres of the
      lateral ligament in the absence of
      bony tenderness (Brooks, Potter and Rainey, 1981)

Tenderness below the lateral malleolus (Vargish et al., 1983)

Ability to weight bear (Vargish et al., 1983)

Some make bold statements: 'Localized tenderness over the anterior fibres of the lateral ligament indicates a partial tear and, in the absence of severe tenderness over the lateral malleolus, may be treated as a simple sprain' (Brooks, Potter and Rainey, 1981). Or 'The absence of moderate tenderness, bruising or swelling in a patient under 61 sustained while walking is a good indication of no bony injury' (Garfield, 1960).

Others quote probabilities, such as patients having tenderness below the lateral malleolus, who are able to weight bear, having a 97.5% probability of a soft tissue injury (Vargish et al., 1983), or the fact that X-raying patients over 60, those with distal fibular tenderness and those unable to weight bear, would pick up 95% of important fractures (Dunlop et al., 1986).

Because no combination of physical findings will predict all injuries, some feel that every injured ankle should be X-rayed (Svenson, 1988). However, assuming that some selection has to be made, the occasional very minor fracture will be missed and, as long as the decision not to X-ray is based on a good (and recorded) physical examination, then no blame should be attached to a doctor who misses such a fracture.

FRACTURES OF THE LATERAL MALLEOLUS

Fractures of the lower third of the fibula may, on occasions, only be seen on the lateral X-ray and, as in this view the fibula is superimposed on the tibia, it may be missed (Figure 17.1). On rare occasions, oblique X-rays may be necessary to demonstrate these better (Figure 17.2).

AVULSION FRACTURES

Small avulsion fractures from the lateral malleolus and talus or, less commonly, the medial malleolus, navicular or other tarsal bones are not significant and do not need specific treatment. It is therefore not

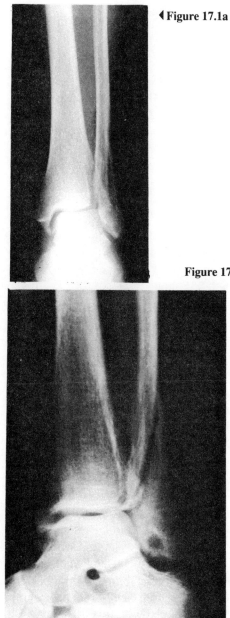

◀ **Figure 17.1a**

Figure 17.1b ▶

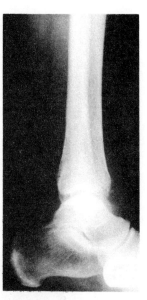

◀ **Figure 17.1c**

Figure 17.1 Fracture lateral malleolus. If the standard X-rays show a possible abnormality whose significance is uncertain, an oblique X-ray may solve the problem.

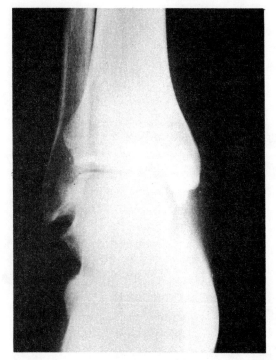

Figure 17.2a

necessary that patients with these injuries are X-rayed but, when an X-ray has been taken, these fractures should be seen although they are frequently missed.

MORE SEVERE ANKLE FRACTURES

It is important that not only is an ankle fracture noted but that its severity and full extent are diagnosed. A fractured lateral malleolus, associated with lateral talar shift (i.e. there is a larger than normal gap between the medial malleolus and the talus), indicates severe ligamentous injury and thus not a simple fracture to be immobilized in plaster but a fracture-dislocation which needs reduction and possible internal fixation.

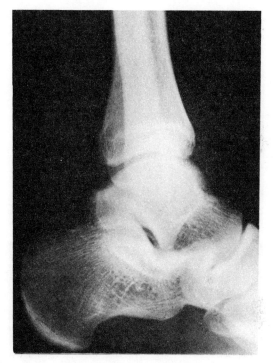

Figure 17.2b

If a patient has lateral talar shift and no fracture of the lateral malleolus, the whole fibula should be examined and X-rayed as, almost certainly, there will be a fracture higher up the fibula.

Fractures of the tibia and fibula may be associated with ankle (particularly posterior malleolar) fractures, which will be missed if not specifically looked for (Van der Werken and Zeegers, 1988).

LIGAMENTOUS INJURIES

The full assessment of a sprained ankle should include stress X-rays of the ankle to exclude ligamentous rupture. However, in the acute situation this may need some form of anaesthesia and will only be

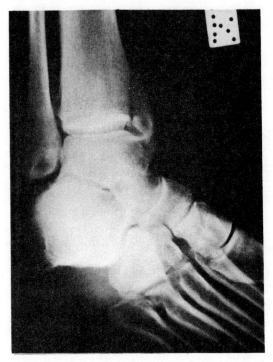

Figure 17.2c

Figure 17.2 Fracture medial malleolus. If the standard X-rays fail to show the injury that you are clinically convinced the patient has, further X-rays, in this case an oblique, may prove your clinical diagnosis correct. Oblique X-rays are useful in other areas of the body, too.

necessary if patient management will be altered. Patients with recurrent sprains should, however, all have stress X-rays.

FRACTURED CALCANEUM

Fractured calcanea are commonly missed injuries, and this occurs because of errors being made at several stages of the diagnostic process. Firstly, the history of a fall onto the heel is not obtained,

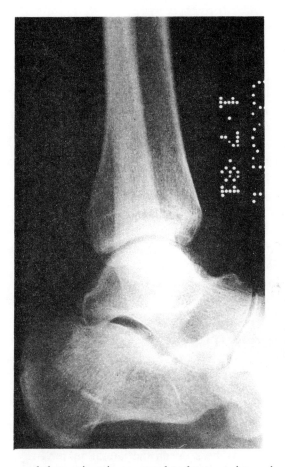

Figure 17.3 Fracture calcaneum. No fracture line is seen but the calcaneum is severely crushed — compare it to Figs 17.1 and 17.2. These injuries are easily missed on ankle X-rays by the inexperienced but it would have been obvious on an axial view of the calcaneum.

and the patient is assumed to have an inversion injury. Palpation for tenderness is therefore restricted to the malleoli and ligaments, and so the acute tenderness of the calcaneum is not found. The doctor asks for ankle X-rays but calcaneal fractures may be difficult to see on standard ankle X-rays (Figure 17.3), and so the injury is missed. If the history had been appreciated, the calcaneal tenderness found and an axial view of the calcaneum obtained, the fracture would have been obvious (Figure 17.3).

Fractures of the calcaneum may be associated with crush fractures of the lumbar spine, and so the back should be examined (and possibly X-rayed) in every case, in order not to miss these associated injuries.

OTHER TARSAL INJURIES

Fractures of the neck of the talus are uncommon but are usually recognized. What may be underestimated is the degree of displacement, with a displaced fracture which needs reduction being thought to be undisplaced.

Some patients with ankle injuries may have *fractures of the cuboid, the navicular or one of the cuneiforms.* These will not be seen on an ankle X-ray and will only be diagnosed on a foot X-ray. While there is usually no specific treatment for these injuries, it is useful to diagnose them so that prolonged pain following an injury can be explained. Foot X-rays should not be done routinely following an ankle injury but should be requested if there is a specific indication.

FRACTURES OF THE FIFTH METATARSAL

Not only may inversion injuries of the ankle cause ankle fractures and sprains, but they may also cause an avulsion fracture at the base of the fifth metatarsal. Occasionally patients suffer both, and the metatarsal fracture is missed while all the attention is directed at the ankle. These injuries need a foot X-ray for their diagnosis but, on occasion, these fractures may be seen on the lateral ankle X-ray, when they are often missed because they are not looked for and the doctor does not go round the edge of every bone with a finger or pen.

MIDTARSAL AND TARSOMETATARSAL (LISFRANC) INJURIES

These injuries are uncommon and, partly for this reason, are not thought of, so are frequently missed (42.8% of midtarsal injuries had a delayed diagnosis in one series) (Main and Jowett, 1975). Inadequate X-rays (Main and Jowett) do not help. The X-ray changes of tarsometatarsal injuries are often not obvious to the inexperienced. 'Routine' foot X-rays in many hospitals consist of an AP and an oblique X-ray, but a lateral X-ray may help. Another factor is that these injuries commonly occur in road accidents when attention is directed at more obvious and serious injuries elsewhere (Hesp, Van der Werken and Goris, 1984).

Ruptured Achilles tendon is a commonly missed injury, and is discussed in Chapter 18.

FALSE POSITIVES

There are a number of radiological variants around the ankle and foot which may cause confusion.

1. Accessory bones. There are numerous accessory bones which may occur around the ankle and foot. These can usually be distinguished from fractures by their characteristic sites and by their smooth, rounded and well corticated appearance, whereas fractures usually have one sharp or jagged edge without a cortex.

    While an accessory bone may be misdiagnosed as a fracture (Griffiths and Menelaus, 1987), it is normally thought to be a minor avulsion fracture requiring no specific treatment, but there is a recorded case of an accessory bone being internally fixed after it had been misdiagnosed as a fracture (Coral, 1986).
2. Old chip and avulsion fractures have similar rounded and corticated appearances.
3. The epiphysis at the base of the fifth metatarsal is frequently mistaken for a fracture, but the epiphyseal plate runs longitudinally whereas fractures at this site run transversely.
4. The epiphysis at the back of the calcaneum is often fragmented.
5. The epiphysis at the base of the proximal phalanx of the big toe may have a longitudinal split in it as a normal variant.
6. There are two sesamoid bones under the head of the first metatarsal. The medial sesamoid is frequently bipartite. This should not be mistaken for a fracture of the sesamoid which can occur but is very rare.

PRACTICAL POINTS

- As always, the history of the mechanism of injury is all important.
- When examining the ankle routinely palpate the calcaneum, the base of the fifth metatarsal and the Achilles tendon, as these are probably the three most commonly missed injuries.
- If your decision on whether to X-ray someone with an ankle injury is based on the criteria in Table 17.1, you will not miss any significant ankle injury.
- If you suspect a fractured calcaneum, always request calcaneal views and, for severe foot injuries, always request a lateral foot X-ray.
- When you look at ankle X-rays, always look for talar shift.

REFERENCES

Brand D.A., Frazier W.H., Kohlhepp W.C. et al. (1982) A protocol for selecting patients with injured extremities who need X-rays. *N. Engl. J. Med.,* **306,** 333–9.

Brooks S.C., Potter B.T. and Rainey J.B. (1981) Inversion injuries of the ankle: clinical assessment and radiographic review. *Br. Med. J.,* **282,** 607–8.

Coral A. (1986) Os subtibiale mistaken for a recent fracture. *Br. Med. J.,* **292,** 1571–2.

Dunlop M.G., Beattie T.F., White G.K.et al. (1986) Guidelines for selective radiological assessment of inversion ankle injuries. *Br. Med. J.,* **293,** 603–5.

Garfield J. (1960) Is radiological assessment of the twisted ankle necessary? *Lancet,* **ii,** 1167–9.

Griffiths J.D. and Menelaus M.B. (1987) Symptomatic ossicles of the lateral malleolus in children. *J. Bone Jt Surg.,* **69B,** 317–9.

Hesp W.L.E.M., Van der Werken C. and Goris R.J.A. (19840 Lisfranc dislocations: Fractures and/or dislocations through the tarso-metatarsal joints. *Injury,* **15,** 261–6.

de Lacey G. and Bradbrooke S. (1979) Rationalising requests for X-ray examination of acute ankle injuries. *Br. Med. J.* **1,** 1597–8.

Main B.J. and Jowett R.L. (1975) Injuries of the midtarsal joint. *J. Bone Jt Surg.,* **57B,** 89–97.

Svenson J. (1988) Need for radiographs in the acutely injured ankle. *Lancet,* **i,** 244–5.

Vargish T., Clarke W.R., Young R.A. et al. (1983) The ankle injury — indications for the selective use of X-rays. *Injury,* **14,** 507–12.

Van der Werken C. and Zeegers E.V.C.M. (1988) Fractures of the lower leg with involvement of the posterior malleolus: a neglected combination. *Injury,* **19,** 241–3.

18 Tendon and nerve injuries

CLOSED TENDON INJURIES

Reasons for misdiagnosis

That these injuries are commonly missed is demonstrated by the fact that many of them have operations well described for the treatment of the late diagnosed case (Editorial, 1980; Lunn and Lamb, 1984). Why are they missed?

The history of something 'giving way' during exertion or a resisted muscle contraction should suggest an injury to a muscle, a tendon or to its attachment to a bone but, with the exception of mallet fingers and ruptured Achilles tendons, they are mostly uncommon injuries. They may thus not even be considered as a cause of the symptoms and not examined for, or the examination on which the diagnosis depends may be inadequate. Occasionally all the abnormal physical signs are described but the diagnosis is missed because the doctor has never heard of the condition: X-rays are normal and the injury is dismissed as 'soft-tissue knee injury' or 'finger injury — X-ray: no bony injury', neither of which is a diagnosis.

Tendon ruptures occur more commonly in patients on steroids and with connective-tissue diseases. In these circumstances the patient may seek help from a physician rather than from an A & E or orthopaedic department, and the possibility of a mechanical cause of what seems to be a flare-up of a systemic disease is not even considered.

Rupture of the central slip of extensor digitorum (boutonnière deformity)

This injury is uncommon, but is commonly (or even usually) missed initially as the inability to fully extend the PIP joint is not noted. It is only when the lateral slips of the tendon move anteriorly and the flexion deformity becomes more severe that the injury is diagnosed.

Flexor tendon ruptures in the hand and forearm

These are uncommon and usually result from hyperextension injuries or flexion against a major force, but they may occur following a crush injury or following an open wound that has partially divided a tendon which ruptures later. A rupture may also occur because of attrition on a rough surface (e.g. following a fracture) (Mahring, Semple and Gray, 1985). The commonest injury is rupture of the flexor digitorum profundus tendon to the ring finger (rugby finger) and this is often missed (Lunn and Lamb, 1984). Rupture of both tendons to a finger has been reported (Mathews and Walton, 1984) and, although functional loss must have been severe, the diagnosis was missed presumably because the possibility of such an injury was never considered. This failure to consider the possibility of such an injury may lead to patients being referred to a neurologist. In a series of 80 flexor tendon ruptures, the authors report 'a few patients had undergone extensive investigations for rare and exotic muscular and nervous disorders before the diagnosis of tendon rupture was considered' (Boyes, Wilson and Smith, 1960).

An example of how a tendon injury can simulate a nerve disorder is the patient with ruptures of flexor pollicis longus and the flexor digitorum profundus tendon to the index finger who was thought to have an anterior interosseous nerve syndrome (Mahring, Semple and Gray, 1985).

Ruptured Achilles tendon

Ruptured Achilles tendon is a fairly common injury but it is still frequently missed, occasionally for months. In one series 20% were missed initially (Inglis et al., 1976). Errors are made at all stages of the diagnostic process.

The history of a sudden onset of pain, such that the patient wonders who hit him, at the back of the heel, which occurs on vigorous exertion (classically running for a bus or playing squash) and sometimes associated with an audible 'snap' virtually gives one the diagnosis if the patient is allowed to give the history or if the doctor listens.

As the most common ankle injury is a sprain, the examination of the ankle is usually directed to the malleoli and ligaments and, if the right history is not obtained, the Achilles tendon may not be palpated for a gap or for tenderness. X-rays, of course, will usually be normal (except in the rare case when there is an avulsion fracture or the tendon is calcified).

Lastly, even if the diagnosis is considered, the fact that the patient can still plantar flex the foot (using the long toe flexors) is often wrongly taken as evidence that the Achilles tendon is intact. The proper examination for a ruptured Achilles tendon, including the gastrocnemius squeeze test (Simmonds' test) needs to be taught and practised. Failure to do this test will lead to a claim for missed diagnosis being indefensible (Thomas, 1986).

Rupture of the extensor mechanism of the knee

Rupture of the quadriceps tendon and the patella ligament are uncommon and are often missed (Editorial, 1980; Siweck and Rao, 1981). In one series, half the quadriceps tendon and more than a quarter of the patella ligament ruptures were initially missed (Siweck and Rao).

The patient with a quadriceps tendon rupture will usually have a palpable gap in the tendon if this is looked for early, but later this may fill with organizing haematoma and become less obvious.

X-rays are normal. Delayed diagnosis leads to poorer results (Siweck and Rao).

Patients with a patella ligament rupture do have an abnormal X-ray but, if the doctor has not considered the diagnosis, he may miss the fact that the unopposed pull of the quadriceps has pulled the patella proximally so that it no longer articulates with the femoral condyles, and dismiss the X-ray as normal.

Diagnosis of both these conditions should be easy if they are considered, as there will be inability to straight leg raise or to extend the knee against gravity. All patients with knee injuries should be instructed on quadriceps exercises and so, even if the diagnosis is initially missed, it should be made when the patient is found to be unable to do these exercises. It should therefore be impossible to miss these injuries! Unfortunately the teaching of quadriceps exercises is not the routine it should be.

Rupture of tibialis posterior

Other closed tendon ruptures in the lower leg are very rare but do occasionally occur and are usually missed (Mann and Thompson, 1985) because the possibility is not considered. Tibialis posterior rupture results in a flat foot.

Muscle tear of gastrocnemius

Patients giving a history similar to that of a ruptured Achilles tendon, but who localize the pain higher in the calf, usually have a tear in the gastrocnemius muscle or musculotendinous junction. The clinical signs may be similar to those of a deep vein thrombosis (DVT) with which it is sometimes confused (occasionally with major consequences, Anouchi, Parker and Seitz, 1987). Usually the history distinguishes between the two but, as leg injury and rest will predispose to DVT, it is not impossible for the two conditions to co-exist, particularly in the patient who develops an exacerbation of symptoms some days after the injury. Venography may be necessary to exclude a DVT in these cases.

Avulsion fractures from the pelvis

Patients with avulsion fractures from the pelvis (e.g. of rectus femoris from the anterior inferior iliac spine) are usually young and give a characteristic history of sudden pain at the height of a sporting activity. These injuries are frequently missed, usually because the diagnosis is not considered.

If the patient is not X-rayed for several weeks, the radiological appearance of healing fracture in a patient, in whom trauma is not considered a cause of symptoms, may be mistaken for a sarcoma.

OPEN TENDON INJURIES

Lacerations of the wrist and hand commonly divide underlying tendons (and nerves). The diagnosis of these depends entirely on the clinical examination. Unfortunately doctors may be unable to test for tendon injuries or may not do it in every case.Tendon injuries are commonly missed and diagnosed late. A primary tendon repair in a patient with a clean wound will frequently give better results than a secondary repair, and so missing a tendon injury deprives a patient of this chance. Having found no tendon injury on examination, it is important that this is recorded, as occasionally tendons may rupture later (either following a crush injury or a partial division) and the doctor may then be falsely accused of missing it.

Tendon injuries around the ankle and foot are less common (as are lacerations in this area) but may have important consequences if undiagnosed and untreated (Citron, 1985). All patients with lacerations of the foot and ankle must have tendon and nerve function tested.

BRACHIAL PLEXUS INJURIES\

Brachial plexus injuries usually occur as a complication of shoulder injuries or as a result of a high velocity injury, and so the patient will almost always have other injuries. If there are significant fractures in the upper limb or if the patient is comatose, it will be more difficult to examine the patient, while if the patient has a head or cervical spine injury, the weakness may be attributed to that. An intravenous infusion sited in a limb may also result in the limb not being properly examined, and for all these reasons brachial plexus injuries are easily overlooked (Grundy and Silver, 1983).

PERIPHERAL NERVE INJURIES

'Early repair of cleanly divided nerves produces the best results' (Birch, 1986). For this reason, if no other, it is important that nerve injuries are diagnosed early but unfortunately '... delay in diagnosis of these injuries is surprisingly common' (Birch). Probably the most commonly missed injury is that of the median nerve, which is more superficial, and thus prone to injury, than many doctors imagine. Digital nerve injuries are also missed and, even if diagnosed, their importance may not be recognized (Finlayson et al., 1986) or the possibility of surgical repair not considered.

Apart from a complete failure to examine the sensation and motor power distal to a wound, the usual cause of missing a nerve injury is to ask the wrong question. To ask 'Can you feel that?' will almost always produce the answer 'Yes', even when the nerve is completed divided. The right question to ask is 'Does that feel normal?' or 'Does it feel the same in all the fingers?' *Altered* sensation within a nerve distribution (or within part of a nerve distribution, as partial lacerations of nerves are not rare) indicates a nerve injury until proved otherwise at surgery.

PRACTICAL POINTS

● It is essential that doctors know how to test for tendon injuries. If you have never been taught, do not try to teach yourself but ask your consultant to teach you.
● There is no excuse for not testing tendon and nerve function distal to every wound.

● Remember that closed tendon ruptures (though uncommon) do occur.

REFERENCES

Anouchi Y.S., Parker R.D. and Seitz W.H. (1987) Anterior compartment syndrome of the calf arising from misdiagnosis of a rupture of the medial head of the gastrocnemius. *J. Trauma*, **27**, 678–80.

Birch R. (1986) Lesions of the peripheral nerves: the present position. *J. Bone Jt Surg.*, **68B**, 2–8.

Boyes J.H., Wilson J.N. and Smith J.W. (1960) Flexor tendon ruptures in the forearm and hand. *J. Bone Jt Surg.*, **42A**, 637–46.

Citron N. (1985) Injury of the tibialis posterior tendon: a cause of acquired valgus foot in childhood. *Injury*, **16**, 610–2.

Editorial (1980) Patella tendon rupture. *Br. Med. J.*, **1**, 1196–7.

Finlayson B.J., Cross A.B., Shalley M.J. et al. (1986) The value of a next day hand injury review clinic. *J. Hand Surg.*, **11B**, 438–40.

Grundy D.J. and Silver J.R. (1983) Combined brachial plexus and spinal cord trauma. *Injury*, **15**, 57–61.

Inglis A.E., Scott W.N., Sculco T.P. et al. (1976) Ruptures of the tendo Achillis. *J. Bone Jt Surg.*, **58A**, 990–3.

Lunn P.G. and Lamb D.W. (1984) Rugby finger — avulsion of profundus of ring finger. *J. Hand Surg.*, **9B**, 69–71.

Mahring M., Semple C. and Gray I.C.M. (1985) Attritional flexor tendon rupture due to a scaphoid non-union imitating an anterior interosseous nerve syndrome. *J. Hand Surg.*, **10B**, 62–4.

Mann R.A. and Thompson F.M. (1985) Rupture of the posterior tibial tendon causing flat foot. *J. Bone Jt Surg.*, **67A**, 556–61.

Mathews R.N. and Walton J.N. (1984) Spontaneous rupture of both flexor tendons in a single digit. *J. Hand Surg.*, **9B**, 134–6.

Siweck C.W. and Rao J.P. (1981) Ruptures of the extensor mechanism of the knee. *J. Bone Jt Surg.*, **63A**, 932–7.

Thomas T.G. (1986) Orthopaedic manholes and rabbit holes: some thoughts on medical negligence. *J. R. Soc. Med.*, **79**, 701–7.

19　Vascular injuries

ARTERIAL INJURIES

Arterial injuries, both open and closed, are important. However, the classical signs of peripheral ischaemia are rare and there are no invariable signs of injury. Common signs of injury are absence of a peripheral pulse, arterial bleeding from a wound, an expanding haematoma and a bruit (Blacklay, Duggan and Wood, 1987). However, injuries do occur in the absence of any of these signs (Thomas and Baird, 1983) and distal pulses may be normal in up to a quarter of patients with peripheral vascular injuries (Blacklay, Duggan and Wood). These injuries are therefore easily missed and a high index of suspicion is essential.

Any wound which, from its position, could have involved an artery, should be assumed to have done so until proved otherwise by a formal surgical exploration or, less commonly, an arteriogram (though even these can be misinterpreted, Feliciano et al., 1984).

Some fractures and dislocations may be complicated by arterial injuries. Although these are uncommon, some associations are listed in Table 19.1. As stated above, there are no invariable signs of arterial injury and, in general, a high index of suspicion and repeated observation is all that is required in these injuries, though some have advocated that routine arteriograms should be done in patients with knee dislocations (McCoy et al., 1987).

Table 19.1 Some bone and joint injuries which may be associated with arterial injury

Injury	Artery
Posterior dislocation sternoclavicular joint	great vessels in neck
Displaced fracture first rib	great vessels in neck
Inferior dislocation of shoulder	axillary
Supracondylar fracture humerus	brachial
Dislocation elbow	brachial
Supracondylar fracture femur	popliteal
Dislocation knee	popliteal

FALSE ANEURYSMS

Open and closed injuries may cause false aneurysms. These are uncommon and, because most of the contents of the aneurysmal sac may consists of clot, they may not be pulsatile. False aneurysms may, therefore, be misdiagnosed as haematomas (Mikulin and Walker, 1984) or even sarcomas if the history of trauma is not appreciated (Gantz, Sweet and Jakim, 1988). Because of the inflammatory response to any injury and the fact that some patients may be pyrexial (Dehne, 1967), a false aneurysm due to open or closed injury may be diagnosed as an abscess (Dehne, 1967; Hueston, 1973; Louis and Simon, 1974; Walsh and Connolly, 1982; Demetriades, Rabinowitz and Sofianos, 1988).

Whether misdiagnosed as a haematoma or an abscess, incision and drainage of a false aneurysm may have the expected disastrous consequences. Before one tries to incise and drain a haematoma, it is wise to try to aspirate it first. This may reveal an aneurysm (Guly, 1986) but, because its contents may be thrombosed, even this is not a diagnostic test.

COMPARTMENT SYNDROMES

A vascular injury of a different type is the compartment syndrome in which increased pressure due to haematoma or swelling within a fascial compartment of a limb reduces capillary perfusion below that necessary for tissue viability, thus causing ischaemic damage to muscle and nerves (of variable degree). These may occur following fractures, vascular injuries, crush injuries and after other soft-tissue injuries and may be very severe in patients with bleeding disorders. The most common symptom and sign is severe pain, especially on stretching the involved muscles. Others include paraesthesiae, paresis, absent pulses (occasionally) and increased tissue pressure when the muscle is palpated. The reliability of these clinical features is debatable, and the only sure way of detecting raised intra-compartmental pressure is to measure it, but this is not routine in most departments (Editorial, 1979). The majority of cases of compartment syndrome are relatively minor and occur following a fracture, and are frequently missed. Departmental guidelines for managing these injuries should take into account the detection of compartment syndromes.

Of more importance is the misdiagnosis of severe compartment syndromes. This may occur in patients, who are unable to feel or complain of pain, e.g. comatose and anaesthetized patients (Macey, 1987) or those with neurological injuries including spinal injury, neuropraxia or even tourniquet paralysis (Luk and Pun, 1987). If the patient has a bony injury or is admitted under an orthopaedic surgeon, the possibility of a compartment syndrome should at least be considered, but this may not happen in patients with soft-tissue injuries (Allen et al., 1985).

PRACTICAL POINTS

- Any wound which could involve an artery should be assumed to have done so until proved otherwise at operation.
- The blood supply should be examined distal to every fracture and every wound. Not only should pulses be palpated but also the temperature, colour, capillary return and whether there is pain on muscle stretching should be observed.
- Before incising a haematoma or an abscess (especially on the buttock) which follows trauma, always consider whether it could be a false aneurysm. Also aspirate it first.

- Patients with crush injuries should be admitted for observation even in the absence of bony injury.
- Any patient whose pain, following either a soft-tissue or bony limb injury, is more severe than you would expect must have a compartment syndrome considered.
- Compartment pressure measurement should be more widely used.

REFERENCES

Allen M.J. Steingold R.F., Kotecha M. et al. (1985) The importance of the deep volar compartment in crush injuries of the forearm. *Injury*, **16**, 273–5.

Blacklay P.F., Duggan E. and Wood R.F.M. (1987) Vascular trauma. *Br. J. Surg.*, **74**, 1077–83.

Dehne E. (1967) Slow arterial leak consequent to unrecognised arterial laceration. *J. Bone Jt Surg.*, **49A**, 372–6.

Demetriades D., Rabinowitz B. and Sofianos C. (1988) Gluteal artery aneurysms. *Br. J. Surg.*, **75**, 494.

Editorial (1979) Muscle compartment syndrome. *Br. Med. J.*, **2**, 818.

Feliciano D.V., Bitondo C.G., Mattox K.L et al. (1984) The missed injury: sins in trauma care. *J. Trauma*, **24**, 657.

Gantz E.D., Sweet M.B.E. and Jakim I. (1988) False aneurysm mimicking an aggressive soft tissue sarcoma. *J. Bone Jt Surg.*, **70A**, 1090–2.

Guly H.R. (1986) Beware the 'haematoma'. *Br. J. Acc.Emerg. Med.*, **1** (June), p. 16.

Hueston J.T. (1973) Traumatic aneurysm of the digital artery. A complication of fasciectomy. *The Hands* **5**, 232–4.

Louis D.S. and Simon M.A. (1974) Traumatic false aneurism of the upper extremity. *J. Bone Jt Surg.*, **56A**, 176–9.

Luk K.D.K. and Pun W.K. (1987) Unrecognised compartmental syndrome in a patient with tourniquet paralysis. *J. Bone Jt Surg.*, **69B**, 97–99.

McCoy G.F., Hannon D.G., Barr R.J. et al. (1987) Vascular injury associated with low-velocity dislocation of the knee. *J. Bone Jt Surg.*, **69B**, 285–7.

Macey A.C. (1987) Compartment syndromes in unconscious patients: a simple aid to diagnosis. *Br. Med. J.*, **294**, 1472–3.

Mikulin T. and Walker E.W. (1984) False aneurysm following blunt trauma. *Injury*, **15**, 309–10.

Thomas W.E.G. and Baird R.N. (1983) Arterial injuries in two Bristol hospitals from 1974–1980. *Injury*, **15**, 30–4.

Walsh M.J. and Conolly W.B. (1982) False aneurysms due to trauma to the hand. *The Hand*, **14**, 177–181.

20   Foreign bodies

FOREIGN BODIES IN WOUNDS

In 1983, 22 missed glass foreign bodies and 27 other missed foreign bodies (e.g. metal, wood, bullets) were reported to the Medical Defence Union (Hawkins, 1985). This must be a very small proportion of all missed foreign bodies, as unfortunately this is a common problem.

Retained glass must be suspected in all lacerations caused by glass and may be missed unless the wound is X-rayed. In one series, of 26 retained glass foreign bodies, 25 were seen on X-ray (Gron, Andersen and Vraa, 1986). The same series also proved that clinical methods are inadequate to exclude a foreign body, as 9 of these patients had had the glass previously missed on wound inspection and probing. Even large pieces of glass may be missed clinically, and metallic foreign bodies may similarly be missed. Very large foreign bodies may also be overlooked on X-ray (Wade, 1985) if they are mistaken for artefacts.

In facial lacerations caused by windscreen glass, as well as removing glass from the wounds, the nose should also be examined because glass foreign bodies lodged in the nostril may be overlooked.

Wood is not radio-opaque, and the diagnosis of a retained wooden foreign body (usually a splinter or thorn) is difficult but important, as it will cause a much greater foreign body reaction than will glass or metal. If a puncture wound was made by a thorn or a pointed object such as a cocktail stick, one should always ask if the point was removed.

When there is uncertainty about the presence of a wooden foreign body, the decision on whether to explore the wound may be difficult, but if it is in a site where infection would have serious consequences (e.g. the palm of the hand), it is vital that the wound is explored, using a tourniquet. This is especially true of blackthorn injuries in the vicinity of joints, as pieces of blackthorn retained in a joint will cause a severe destructive arthritis.

A puncture wound which becomes infected usually indicates a retained foreign body and so should be explored and not treated with antibiotics (Rand, 1987).

It should not be forgotten that a stab or other penetrating wound through clothing or a puncture wound through a shoe (e.g. standing on a nail) may cause a piece of clothing or shoe leather to be retained in the depth of the wound, where its presence is not considered until the wound becomes infected (Evans and Ryan, 1987). These wounds should be explored and left open.

Practical points

- *All* wounds caused by broken glass should be X-rayed.
- When you request an X-ray to exclude a foreign body, state this on the form, as the X-ray will be done using a different exposure from that required for diagnosing fractures.
- Always mark the point of entry or the point of maximum tenderness before obtaining an X-ray, as this will assist in localizing the foreign body. If it is not done, the X-rays will need to be repeated with a marker before surgery anyway.
- A puncture or penetrating wound that becomes infected should be surgically explored and not just treated with antibiotics.

INTRA-OCULAR FOREIGN BODIES

About six cases of missed intra-ocular foreign bodies are reported to the Medical Defence Union every year (Hawkins, 1985). As with so many injuries, it is the history which suggests the diagnosis, and poor history taking will lead to the diagnosis not being considered.

A history that a patient has been 'hit in the eye' needs elaboration, as a blow with a large, blunt object will cause different injuries from those caused by a small piece of stone or steel shot into the eye while chiselling. The latter history should always suggest a foreign body and, if no foreign body is found on the cornea or on the conjunctiva, it should be assumed to be in the globe, and the patient should be X-rayed. Perforating wounds of the cornea or sclera should also suggest the possibility of an intra-ocular foreign body.

Practical point

● If there is any possibility of an intra-ocular foreign body, the eye *must* be X-rayed.

FOREIGN BODIES IN THE RESPIRATORY AND ALIMENTARY TRACTS

These usually present to A & E departments with a history of possible ingestion or aspiration of a foreign body, and this chapter is devoted to misdiagnosis in this setting. It must also be realised that, especially in children, there may be no history and so a foreign body may be overlooked as a cause of chronic symptoms. This is not an acute problem and so, apart from advising that a foreign body should always be considered as a cause for the unexplained nasal discharge or the unexplained lung collapse, I will not further discuss these problems.

Fish bones stuck in the throat

Many patients attend A & E departments with a feeling that something has stuck in their throats but, as only a minority (though a substantial one) turn out to have a foreign body, the seriousness of the problem may not be realized, so that the fish bones may be missed which will cause infection and possibly death (Kirkham and English, 1984).

163

The only safe way to approach this problem is to assume that every patient who thinks he has a bone stuck does have one until it can be proved that this is not so.

Firstly, the oropharynx should be carefully examined, especially the tonsillar beds, to ensure that there is nothing there.

Secondly the patient should be X-rayed. About 75% of fish bones should be visible on a good quality X-ray (Kirkham and English) but it is important that it is of good quality and that, as on an X-ray taken for trauma, one can see all seven cervical vertebrae. Soft-tissue swelling, air in the soft tissues and air trapped in the oesophagus round a foreign body should be looked for. If the laryngeal cartilages are calcified, the X-ray will be more difficult to interpret, but repeating the X-ray while the patient does a Valsalva manoeuvre will cause a cartilaginous opacity to move, whereas a foreign body will stay put (Hadley, 1984).

Next, all patients should have an indirect laryngoscopy. If the patient has a normal X-ray and a normal indirect laryngoscopy and if his symptoms are slight (e.g. he can eat and drink normally), he can be discharged but with instructions to return if symptoms do not improve over 24 hours.

If he has significant symptoms, he should be referred to an ENT surgeon for consideration for endoscopy.

Inhaled foreign body

The acute complete obstruction of the upper airway with food is a cause of sudden unexpected death (Mittleman and Wetli, 1982) and needs to be recognized immediately at the scene of the incident so that the food can be expelled, using the Heimlich manoeuvre (1983). Failure to diagnose the condition will be fatal.

Inhaled foreign bodies which present to the A & E department are usually smaller and lodge further down the respiratory tract. The diagnosis is frequently delayed and this increases the risk of complications (Esclamado and Richardson, 1987). Inhaled foreign bodies are most common in children and in adults with swallowing disorders. If a denture of a patient with a swallowing disorder, or who is unconscious, is found to be missing (Valori and Leclerc, 1985), the possibility of its being in the respiratory tract should be considered, and missing teeth or dentures in patients with facial injuries may be lodged there too.

In most cases a history of aspiration or choking suggests the diagnosis, and the acute onset of stridor or wheezing in appropriate circumstances is also suggestive (Esclamado and Richardson). Neck X-rays may suggest the presence of laryngeal and tracheal foreign bodies but initial chest X-rays may be normal (Esclamado and Richardson), though a chest X-ray taken in expiration may show air trapping (Griffiths and Freeman, 1984). The secret of correctly diagnosing these foreign bodies is that, once the possibility of a foreign body has been raised, the diagnosis should be assumed until proved otherwise. The only sure investigation is endoscopy.

The causes of failing to diagnose inhaled (and ingested) foreign bodies have been summarized as: failure to consider the possibility; failure to elicit the history; the absence of history; scepticism of the possibility of a foreign body; an apathetic attitude of the doctor; a symptomless interval; multiplicity of foreign bodies; awaiting spontaneous expulsion; symptoms explained by other medical conditions; lack of emphasis in medical teaching; and the character of the foreign body (Bradley and Narula, 1984).

Practical point

● If a patient says a fish bone is stuck in the throat, or once the possibility of an inhaled foreign body has been raised, it should be assumed to be present until appropriate investigations have proved otherwise.

Swallowed foreign bodies

Children very commonly swallow small objects, and the vast majority of these pass through the alimentary tract without causing problems but larger foreign bodies, such as coins, may impact in the oesophagus. Whereas these usually causes pain, dysphagia and drooling, it may be asymptomatic (Hashemi and Harvey, 1987; Holborn and Da Cruz, 1987). As this is clearly an important diagnosis which should not be missed, any child who has ingested an object large enough to impact should (if the object is radio-opaque) be X-rayed to exclude impaction.

If chest and abdominal X-rays fail to show the unexpected foreign body, it may be lodged in the nasopharynx (Parker, Bingham and Osborne, 1988).

REFERENCES

Bradley P.J. and Narula A. (1984) 'I have a bone stuck in my throat'. *Br. Med. J.,* **289,** 761.

Esclamado R.M. and Richardson M.A. (1987) Laryngotracheal foreign bodies in children. *Am. J. Dis. Child.,* **141,** 259–62.

Evans P.D. and Ryan P. (1987) Penetrating injuries of the scrotum association with later abdominal wall abscesses. *J. R. Coll. Surg. Edinb.,* **32,** 111.

Griffiths D.M. and Freeman N.V. (1984) Expiratory chest X-ray examination in the diagnosis of inhaled foreign bodies. *Br. Med. J.,* **288,** 1074–5.

Gron P., Andersen K. and Vraa A. (1986) Detection of glass foreign bodies by radiography. *Injury,* **17,** 404–6.

Hadley M.D.M. (1984) 'I have a bone stuck in my throat'. *Br. Med. J.,* **289,** 761–2.

Hashemi K. and Harvey K. (1987) 'Hunt the thimble': a study of the radiology of ingested foreign bodies. *Arch. Emerg. Med.,* **4,** 197.

Hawkins C. (1985) *Mishap or Malpractice,* Oxford, Blackwell Scientific Publications, pp. 137–42.

Heimleich H.J. (1983) The Heimlich manoeuvre. *Br. Med. J.,* **286,** 1349–50.

Holborn C. and Da Cruz D. (1987) 'Hunt the thimble': a study of the radiology of ingested foreign bodies. *Arch. Emerg. Med.,* **4,** 197–8.

Kirkham N. and English R. (1984) 'I have a bone stuck in my throat'. *Br. Med. J.,* **289,** 424–5.

Mittleman R.E. and Wetli C.V. (1982) The fatal cafe coronary: foreign body airway obstruction. *JAMA,* **247,** 1285–8.

Parker A.J., Bingham B.J. and Osborne J.E. (1988) 'The swallowed foreign body: is it in the nasopharynx?' *Postgrad. Med. J.,* **64,** 201–3.

Rand C. (1987) Cocktail stick injuries: delayed diagnosis of a retained foreign body. *Br. Med. J.,* **295,** 1658.

Valori R.M. and Leclerc J. (1985) Impacted dentures mimicking brain stem stroke in a conscious patient. *Br. Med. J.,* **290,** 1413–4.

Wade P.J.F. (1985) Penetrating injury of the thigh: a missed radiological diagnosis. *Injury,* **16,** 568–9.

21   Other conditions

BURNS

There is usually no difficulty about diagnosing a burn though, in the context of children with suspected non-accidental injury, impetigo may be misdiagnosed as cigarette burns, and abrasions, chilblains, napkin dermatitis and fixed drug eruption have all been misdiagnosed as burns (Wheeler and Hobbs, 1988). Toxic epidermal necrolysis (staphylococcal scalded skin syndrome) and epidermolysis bullosa may also be confused with scalds.

However, it is common to misdiagnose the depth of a burn and also to fail to recognize the symptoms and signs of inhalational burns until the patient has severe airway or respiratory problems. These are shown in Table 21.1.

Table 21.1 Evidence suggestive of an inhalational burn or smoke inhalation

1. Circumstances of burn
    exposure in an enclosed space
    unconsciousness or inebriation associated with smoke inhalation
    fires involving plastics
    steam inhalation

2. Clinical features
    facial burns
    singeing of nasal hairs
    soot in the nose or mouth or soot in the sputum
    tachypnoea, cough, hoarseness, stridor, wheezing, dyspnoea

It is also very common to misdiagnose the size of a burn, sometimes by as much as 100% (Hammond and Ward, 1987) which will have major implications when calculating fluid replacement volumes. This is usually an overestimation and is often accounted for by including the erythema in the size of the burn, whereas the size should describe only the area of partial thickness and deep burn. Another factor may be that the casualty officer tends to describe the size of a burn at the level which he knows the burns unit will have no choice but to admit! It is essential to use the Lund–Browder or similar charts to estimate burn size.

NEAR DROWNING

Near drowning is usually readily diagnosed by the circumstances in which the patient has been found. However, the reason why the patient came to be in the water needs to be considered (Editorial, 1981) as otherwise underlying conditions, such as myocardial infarction or head injury, may be overlooked.

In temperate parts of the world, near drowning is frequently associated with hypothermia, which should be looked for. This may mimic death. Hypothermia (and possibly other factors) protect the patient against the effects of hypoxia, such that some patients have been successfully resuscitated after 40 or more minutes of submersion (Pearn, 1985). Near drowning and hypothermia causing a lowered level of consciousness, arreflexia and pupillary dilatation may rarely mimic a head injury (Todd and Conn, 1988).

Diving, whether from a board, or from the beach into surf, may cause a cervical spine injury which must not be overlooked in a near drowned patient (Pearn, 1985; Morgan and Winter, 1986).

DECOMPRESSION SICKNESS

Decompression sickness in divers or pressure workers may present as either pain in joints (the bends) or as neurological disease (either intracranial or spinal). This is very uncommon in most A & E departments, and so the diagnosis may be overlooked or even denied by the doctor if the patient suggests is (Wilmshurst, 1988). As the onset of symptoms may be delayed following a dive, it is vital that decompression sickness is considered as a cause of any symptoms coming on within 36 hours of a dive, and that appropriate advice is sought.

Practical points

- Always calculate burn areas using a Lund–Browder chart.
- Drowned and hypothermic patients who seem clinically dead may be capable of resuscitation. Death in these patients can only be diagnosed if one fails to resuscitate them once their body temperature has been restored to normal.
- Consider decompression sickness as a cause for *any* symptoms coming on within 36 hours of diving.

REFERENCES

Editorial (1981) Immersion or drowning. *Br. Med. J.,* **282,** 1340–1.

Hammond J.S. and Ward C.G. (1987) Transfers from emergency room to burn center: errors in burn size estimate. *J. Trauma,* **27,** 1161–5.

Morgan G.A.R. and Winter R.J. (1986) Drowning and near drowning. *Br. Med. J.,* **293,** 395.

Pearn J. (1985) The management of near drowning. *Br. Med. J.,* **291,** 1447–52.

Todd N.V. and Conn A. (1986) Near drowning and hypothermia mimicking severe closed head injury. *Br. Med. J.,* **293,** 594–5.

Wheeler D. and Hobbs C.J. (1988) Mistakes in diagnosing non-accidental injury: 10 years' experience. *Br. Med. J.,* **296,** 1233–6.

Wilmshurst P. (1988) The bends. *Br. Med. J.,* **297,** 916.

22   Multiple injuries

INTRODUCTION

If a patient has an obvious injury, it is very common for both doctor and patient to overlook a less obvious and less painful (though possibly more serious) injury elsewhere.

Retrospective studies of trauma deaths (Hoffman, 1976; Moylan et al., 1976; West, Trunkey and Lim, 1979; Dove, Stahl and del Guercio, 1980; Gilroy, 1984; Kreis et al., 1986; Anderson et al., 1988) have shown that a significant percentage of trauma deaths in hospital are preventable and, in a large proportion of these, a missed or delayed diagnosis was a major cause (Table 22.1).

Other series, looking at all patients with injuries, not just fatal ones, have also shown a large percentage of injuries to be missed. The incidence of missed injuries has been reported as 7.5% (Pringle, 1973), 12% (Chan, Ainscow and Sikorski, 1980), 20.8% (Trinca, 1982) and 38.1% (including false positives) (McClaren, Robertson and Little, 1983). These are injuries of all severities, both bony and soft tissue.

That life-threatening injuries should not be missed is obvious, but it is also important not to miss what may seem to be a very minor injury. In a patient with a ruptured spleen and a flail chest, a dislocated finger will not be a priority, but it is essential that it is not overlooked as, while the patient may make a full recovery from the major injuries, a finger dislocation undiagnosed and untreated for several weeks may cause permanent disability. Delays in diagnosis may also lead to patients requiring additional general anaesthetics (Pringle, 1973).

Table 22.1 Commonest missed diagnoses contributing to avoidable death in 170 hospital trauma deaths (Anderson et al., 1988)

Head and neck	
intracranial haematoma	14
lacerated neck vessel	3
cervical spine fracture	2
Thorax	
lung laceration	18
haemothorax	6
pneumothorax	3
subclavian artery laceration	2
Abdomen	
ruptured liver	22
ruptured spleen	12
ruptured mesentery	7
ruptured kidney	5
ruptured pancreas	3
perforated small bowel	3
perforated bladder	3
perforated ulcer	3
ruptured diaphragm	2
lacerated iliac vessels	2

Specific situations in which injuries are missed are discussed later, but general factors identified as causing missed diagnoses are: inexperience (Dearden and Rutherford, 1985), poor physical examination (Dearden and Rutherford), failure to interpret clinical information (Chan, Ainscow and Sikorski, 1980), failure to X-ray (Chan, Ainscow and Sikorski, 1980; McClaren, Robertson and Little, 1983), poor quality X-rays (Chan, Ainscow and Sikorski, 1980) and mis-interpretation of X-rays (Chan, Ainscow and Sikorski, 1980; McClaren, Robertson and Little, 1983). Finally, the chance of rectifying diagnostic errors made in the A & E department will be lessened if X-ray reports are not read or if the patient is admitted to an inappropriate ward (Chan, Ainscow and Sikorski, 1980; Hamdan, 1987).

INJURIES ASSOCIATED WITH HEAD INJURIES

Head-injured patients will frequently have associated injuries which are frequently overlooked (Irving and Irving, 1976). The main reasons for this are the difficulties of communicating with and examining a patient with a diminished level of consciousness, and also because the doctor concentrates on the head injury (which may seem the major problem) and ignores the rest of the body. This is dangerous, not only because of the risks of death and morbidity due to the injuries missed, but also because the optimum management of the head injury involves maintaining the patient's general state (e.g. oxygenation and haemodynamics). Thus excessive concentration on an injured head is not only bad patient management but it is also bad head injury management.

Spinal injuries

Head injuries are very commonly associated with spinal injuries, and the latter may be overlooked (Ravichandran and Silver, 1982; Shalley and Cross, 1984; Reid et al., 1987) not only because of the difficulties caused by a lowered level of consciousness, but also because neurological signs caused by the spinal injury may be attributed to the head injury.

Apart from bruising or deformity of the spine, other signs which indicate a spinal cord injury in the presence of a severe head injury are (Harris, 1968):

1. Absent intercostal breathing (in cervical cord injuries)
2. Priapism
3. Absence of sweating below the lesion
4. A discrepancy between a patient's response to pain at different levels, e.g. if a patient grimaces to a painful stimulus applied to the face but there is no response to one applied to the arms or legs, this may indicate a tetraplegia, whereas a discrepancy between arms and legs may indicate a paraplegia.

If a patient with a head injury is to be treated with positive pressure ventilation, it is vital that the patient is examined

173

neurologically beforehand, as it will be impossible to do so once he has been given muscle relaxants. If possible, the cervical spine should be X-rayed before intubation.

Chest injuries

The head-injured patient is usually nursed supine, and this makes the interpretation of chest X-rays for pneumothorax and haemothorax very difficult (Chapter 9).

Abdominal injuries

Physical examination of the abdomen in the comatose head-injured patient is very difficult, and may be impossible to interpret, as tenderness cannot be elicited and abdominal wall rigidity is much less common in patients with abdominal injury associated with head injury than in patients without head injury (Wilson, Vidrine and Rives, 1965). If abdominal rigidity is present, it is not caused by the head injury unless the limbs are also held rigid (Wilson, Vidrine and Rives) and neither should a paralytic ileus be attributed to a head injury. Shock in a head-injured patient is almost always due to other injuries (Illingworth and Jennett, 1965; Wilson, Vidrine and Rives, 1965; Butterworth et al., 1980) and, in the absence of any evidence of blood loss elsewhere, intra-abdominal bleeding must always be considered.

Any patient with a head injury, in whom intra-abdominal injury cannot definitely be excluded, must be further investigated with peritoneal lavage (Butterworth et al., 1980) or some other method (Chapter 10).

INJURIES ASSOCIATED WITH SPINAL INJURIES AND OTHER CAUSES OF SENSORY LOSS

Patients with spinal cord injuries will not complain of pain distal to the level of injury. Although limb injuries should be diagnosed by physical examination and X-rays, abdominal injuries may be impossible to diagnose clinically. Not only are they easily missed (Jaffray, Jones and Pringle, 1985) because there will be no pain and physical examination of a flaccid abdominal wall will detect no tenderness or guarding, but they may also be overdiagnosed, as the hypotension and paralytic ileus which accompanies tetraplegia and paraplegia may be assumed to be due to intra-abdominal injury. It is therefore essential that every patient with a spinal injury, in whom an intra-abdominal injury is a possibility, must have further investigation of the abdomen by peritoneal lavage (Tibbs et al., 1980) or some other method (Chapter 10).

Brachial plexus injury in a patient with a spinal cord injury may be overlooked if the weakness is attributed to the cord injury.

Other causes of sensory loss following injury such as plexus or peripheral nerve injury will also mask the pain of injuries and complications such as compartment syndromes, causing difficulty in their diagnosis (Luk and Pun, 1987).

Not only is diagnosis difficult in patients with an acute injury, but injuries (and other problems) may be difficult to diagnose in patients with longstanding spinal cord and other problems (Chapter 4).

The fact that a patient may have more than one spinal fracture and the misdiagnosis of these has been described in Chapter 7.

MORE THAN ONE INJURY IN ONE LIMB

A fall on the outstretched hand may cause one of a number of injuries, including Colles fracture, scaphoid fracture and radial head fracture. Uncommonly a patient may have more than one fracture (Cooney, Dobyns and Linscheid, 1980; Funk and Wood, 1988; Smith et al., 1988) and when this occurs the more obvious injury will be diagnosed, and the less obvious one may be missed (Cooney, Dobyns and Linscheid).

Similarly an inversion injury to the ankle may cause a fractured base of fifth metatarsal as well as an ankle sprain or fracture, and it is very easy for this to be overlooked.

Multiple fractures in a hand or foot are common and so, when an X-ray of hand, foot (or any other part of the body) is looked at, it is important that, even if a fracture is found, the whole X-ray should be looked at and the edge of every bone on the X-ray gone round with a finger or pencil, as otherwise fractures may be missed (Guly, 1984; Juhl and Saether, 1987).

If the limb fracture is a more serious one, diagnosis of other injuries in the limb may be even more difficult, as it may be impossible to move the limb and thus examine for other fractures and possibly nerve injuries. In addition, the classical deformity of one injury may be masked by other displaced fractures in the same limb. In the presence of one serious injury to a limb, it is very common for another injury (usually a more proximal one) to be missed. Thus a posterior hip dislocation (Helal and Skevis, 1967) or a femoral neck fracture (Shaheen and Badr, 1987) may be missed in association with femoral shaft fracture or other lower limb injury (Nixon, 1976), and a dislocation of the shoulder may be overlooked if it is in the same limb as a fractured shaft of humerus (Barquet et al., 1985).

COMMON ASSOCIATIONS OF INJURIES

The common association between a head injury and a cervical spine injury and the less common association between a fractured shaft of femur and a dislocated hip have been discussed above, but there are

Table 22.2 Common associations of injuries

Fractured calcaneum	crush fracture lumbar spine
Knee injuries (in road accident)	dislocation hip
Fractured first rib	brachial plexus and subclavian artery injury (Phillips, Rogers and Gaspar, 1981)
Fractured lower ribs	liver, spleen injury
Fractured sternum	mediastinal injury
Spiral fracture lower tibia	fracture upper fibula

other situations in which an easily diagnosed injury may be associated with another injury which is both more serious and more difficult to diagnose. Some of these are listed in Table 22.2. These associations must be considered whenever the injury is seen, otherwise the more serious condition may be overlooked.

In addition, an injuring force tends to injure adjacent parts of the body. Thus, if two parts of the body have obvious injuries, it is probable that any part in between has also been injured. Thus a patient with a chest injury and a pelvic injury is highly likely to have an abdominal injury as well, or a patient, in whom one can demonstrate upper rib fractures and lower rib fractures on the same side, has probably also fractured the ribs in the middle.

BILATERAL INJURIES

Clinical teachers frequently imply that the only reason that a person is born with two arms and two legs is to assist the doctor who has to examine a diseased or injured part by allowing comparison with the uninjured side.

This is usually of immense value, but the doctor comes unstuck when both sides are injured, as bilateral injuries seem more likely to be missed than unilateral ones. Not only are there difficulties in examining these patients, but bilateral injuries may simulate other diseases. In addition, bilateral shoulder and hip injuries may be caused by seizures which may not be thought of as a cause of bony injury.

Shoulder dislocations

If unilateral shoulder dislocations (especially posterior dislocations) can be missed (Chapter 11), it is hardly surprising that a large proportion of bilateral dislocations are also missed (McFie, 1976; Brown, 1984; Karpinski and Porter, 1984). The patient who is unable to move either arm following an injury may be misdiagnosed for months as having a partial cervical cord injury, and thus have the neck X-rayed rather than the shoulders (personal knowledge).

Hip fractures

A patient with bilateral hip fractures, initially diagnosed as having a neurological deficit, has been reported (McGlone and Gosnold, 1987). More specifically, bilateral hip fractures may simulate paraplegia (personal knowledge).

Quadriceps tendon rupture

Unilateral quadriceps tendon ruptures are frequently missed (Chapter 18). Bilateral rupture does occur and, not surprisingly, is also often missed and may be diagnosed as a stroke (MacEacher and Plewes, 1984), acute rheumatoid arthritis (Preston and Adicoff, 1962) and osteoarthritis (Dahr, 1988).

Achilles tendon rupture

A patient who was eventually diagnosed as having bilateral Achilles tendon ruptures has been reported (Dickey and Patterson, 1987). She presented with a sudden onset of unsteadiness of gait, diminished power of ankle flexion and absent ankle jerks, which simulated an acute peripheral neuropathy.

Bilateral patella ligament rupture

In patients with systemic diseases, tendon ruptures may occur insidiously rather than as an acute injury. A patient with SLE, with an insidious onset of bilateral patella ligament rupture, was initially thought to have a steroid myopathy (Cooney, Aversa and Newman, 1980).

INJURIES MIMICKING OTHER CONDITIONS

Bilateral injuries mimicking other injuries or even non-traumatic conditions have been described above, and the misdiagnosis which may occur when there is no history of trauma are also mentioned elsewhere, but other patterns of injury may mimic other conditions. The following are two cases from the author's experience.

1. An elderly woman fell in an old people's home, and was diagnosed by her general practitioner as having a right hemiplegia. Four days later, she was referred to hospital, where she was discovered to have a fractured surgical neck of her right humerus, a fractured neck of her right femur and an old fractured right olecranon.
2. A 19-year-old boy fell from a cliff, sustaining multiple injuries, including a head injury and a paraplegia. An ipsilateral facial nerve palsy and brachial plexus injury were initially misdiagnosed as being a hemiplegia due to the head injury.

DIAGNOSTIC ERRORS DURING RESUSCITATION

All resuscitation, including that of the seriously injured, is based on the correct management of the airway, the breathing and the circulation. Mismanagement of each of these occurs in patients with severe injuries (Dearden and Rutherford, 1985) and contributes towards trauma deaths (Hoffman, 1976; Moylan et al., 1976; Rose, Valtonen and Jennett, 1977; Yates, 1977; Dove, Stahl and del Guercio, 1980; Anderson et al., 1988). Even if not fatal, it may contribute to a shock lung and other organ failures and may adversely affect the prognosis of head injuries.

Mismanagement may occur because an inexperienced doctor is unable to do a procedure (e.g. insertion of a chest drain, Dearden and Rutherford, 1985) or endotracheal intubation, but more often occurs because airway obstruction, breathing difficulties and hypovolaemia are not diagnosed. When discussing diagnostic errors in the multiply injured, it is important briefly to discuss these errors of diagnosing physiology as well as misdiagnosis of specific anatomical injuries.

Airway obstruction

Airway obstruction is very common in patients with multiple injuries, especially in the situations listed in Table 22.3. In all these situations, airway obstruction should be assumed to be present and every effort made to keep the airway patent. If a patient can tolerate an endotracheal tube, he should be intubated, and the patient who will not tolerate it may also need intubation, in which case he needs to be paralysed and sedated. The fact that an endotracheal tube is in place does not guarantee a clear airway, as it is not unknown for tubes to kink or to become displaced, nor will a tube prevent the patient from drowning in blood produced in the lungs from a ruptured bronchus or a lung contusion.

Table 22.3 Injuries in which airway problems can be predicted

Coma of any cause
Middle third facial fractures
Bilateral mandibular fractures
Soft tissue injuries of the tongue and mouth
Any cause of bleeding into the pharynx in a comatose patient
Laryngeal injury
Chest injuries with haemoptysis
Inhalational burns

Breathing problems

Ventilatory problems too can be predicted from the injuries that the patient has suffered (Table 22.4). It is essential that the adequacy of ventilation is monitored by measurement of arterial blood gases at regular intervals in all significantly injured patients, and that ventilation is maintained by artificial ventilation if necessary.

Table 22.4 Situations in which breathing problems can be anticipated

Airway problems of any kind (see Table 22.3)
Aspiration
Chest injuries including flail chest, lung contusion, pneumothorax,
    haemothorax and diaphragmatic hernia
Head injuries causing hypoventilation
Cervical cord injuries causing loss of intercostal respiration
Pre-existing chest diseases

These are all made worse by abdominal injury or abdominal
distension causing splinting of the diaphragm.

Blood loss

Blood loss is commonly underestimated, leading to inadequate fluid replacement. The reason for this is the poor understanding of physiology that expects the blood pressure to fall and the pulse rate to rise in proportion to the blood loss. This neglects the compensatory mechanisms which aim to maintain cardiac output. In fact, one needs to lose 20% of one's blood volume before the blood pressure starts to fall, and frequently major blood loss will cause the heart rate to fall due to vagal activity (Sander-Jensen et al., 1986).

The shocked patient will be pale, sweating, anxious, hyperventilating and will have cold extremities, and these signs should be looked for and treated as evidence that the patient's cardiovascular system is compensating for blood loss, even if the pulse and blood pressure are normal.

The volume of fluid replacement in the injured patient should be based on the estimated blood loss calculated from the diagnosed injuries, and should not be based on the pulse rate and blood pressure. Clinical signs of shock, as above, should be regarded as evidence that there is still fluid depletion. Central venous pressure measurement should be commenced as soon as practicable.

Practical points

- In all injured patients, examine the joint above and the joint below any obvious injury.
- Any patient involved in a road accident or fall should be examined from head to toe.
- In any injured patient who is admitted to hospital, this head to toe examination should be repeated the following day and probably at intervals until the patient is discharged.
- The cervical spine should be X-rayed routinely in all patients unconscious from a head injury.
- In the seriously injured patient, it may be necessary to delay some non-essential X-rays until the patient's condition has stabilized. If this is done, it must be noted and the X-rays done later.

● Abdominal injuries may be impossible to diagnose in patients with head injuries and spinal injuries. If there is any possibility of abdominal injury, it must be excluded with peritoneal lavage, ultrasound or CT.

● All patients with serious leg injuries should have an X-ray of the pelvis, and all patients with a serious injury in one limb should have the whole limb X-rayed.

● All patients with multiple injuries must have a chest X-ray and a pelvic X-ray.

REFERENCES

Anderson I.D., Woodford M., de Dombal F.T. et al. (1988) Retrospective study of 1,000 deaths from injury in England and Wales. *Br. Med. J.*, **296**, 1305–8.

Barquet A., Schimchak M., Carreras O. et al. (1985) Dislocation of the shoulder with fracture of the ipsilateral shaft of the humerus. *Injury*, **16**, 300–2.

Brown R.J. (1984) Bilateral dislocation of the shoulder. *Injury*, **15**, 267–73.

Butterworth J.F., Maull K.I., Miller J.D. et al. (1980) Detection of occult abdominal trauma in patients with severe head injuries. *Lancet*, **ii**, 759–62.

Chan R.N.W., Ainscow D. and Sikorski J.M. (1980) Diagnostic failures in the multiply injured. *J. Trauma*, **20**, 684–7.

Cooney L.M., Aversa J.M. and Newman J.H. (1980) Insidious bilateral infrapatellar tendon rupture in a patient with systemic lupus erythematosus. *Ann. Rheum. Dis.*, **39**, 592–95.

Cooney W.P., Dobyns J.H. and Linscheid R.L. (1980) Complications of Colles fracture. *J. Bone Jt Surg.*, **62A**, 613–9.

Dearden C.H. and Rutherford W.J. (1985) The resuscitation of the severely injured in the accident and emergency department — a medical audit. *Injury*, **16**, 249–52.

Dhar S. (1988) Bilateral simultaneous spontaneous rupture of the quadriceps tendon. A report of 3 cases and review of the literature. *Injury*, **19**, 7–8.

Dickey W. and Patterson V. (1987) Bilateral Achilles tendon rupture simulating peripheral neuropathy: unusual complication of steroid therapy. *J. R. Soc. Med.*, **80**, 386–7.

Dove D.B., Stahl W.M. and del Guercio L.R.M. (1980) A five year review of deaths following urban trauma. *J. Trauma*, **20**, 760–6.

Funk D.A. and Wood M.B. (1988) Concurrent fractures of the ipsilateral scaphoid and radial head. *J. Bone Jt Surg.*,**70A**, 134–6.

Gilroy D. (1984) Deaths from blunt trauma: a review of 105 cases. *Injury*, **15**, 304–8.

Guly H.R. (1984) Missed diagnoses in an accident and emergency department. *Injury*, **15**, 403–6.

Hamdan T.A. (1987) Missed injuries in casualties from the Iraqi-Iranian war: a study of 35 cases. *Injury,* **18,** 15–17.

Harris P. (1968) Associated injuries in traumatic paraplegia and tetraplegia. *Paraplegia,* **5,** 215–20.

Helal B. and Skevis X. (1967) Unrecognised dislocation of the hip in fractures of the femoral shaft. *J. Bone Jt Surg.,* **49B,** 293–300.

Hoffman E. (1976) Mortality and morbidity following road accidents. *J. R. Coll. Surg. Engl.,* **58,** 233–40.

Illingworth G. and Jennett W.B. (1965) The shocked head injury. *Lancet,* **ii,** 511–4.

Irving M.H. and Irving P.M. (1976) Associated injuries in head injured patients. *J. Trauma,* **7,** 500–11.

Jaffray D.C., Jones H.W.F. and Pringle R.G. (1985) Renal pelvi-uretic injury in traumatic paraplegia. *Injury,* **16,** 244–6.

Juhl M. and Saether J. (1987) Simultaneous dislocation of the interphalangeal joint of the thumb and the carpal lunate. *J. Trauma,* **27,** 581–2.

Karpinski M.R.K. and Porter K.M. (1984) Two cases of bilateral posterior dislocation of the shoulder. *Injury,* **15,** 274–6.

Kreis D.J., Plasencia G., Augenstein D. et al (1986) Preventable trauma deaths: Dade County, Florida. *J. Trauma,* **26,** 649–54.

Luk K.D.K. and Pun W.K. (1987) Unrecognised compartmental syndrome in a patient with tourniquet paralysis. *J. Bone Jt Surg.,* **69B,** 97–99.

McClaren C.A.N., Robertson C. and Little K. (1983) Missed orthopaedic injuries in the resuscitation room. *J. R. Coll. Surg. Edinb.,* **28,** 399–401.

MacEacher A.G. and Plewes J.L. (1984) Bilateral simultaneous spontaneous rupture of the quadriceps tendons. 5 case reports and a review of the literature. *J. Bone Jt Surg.,* **66B,** 81–3.

McFie J. (1976) Bilateral anterior dislocation of the shoulders. A case report. *Injury,* **8,** 67–9.

McGlone R. and Gosnold J.K. (1987) Posterior dislocation of the shoulder and bilateral hip fractures caused by epileptic seizure. *Arch. Emerg. Med.,* **4,** 115–6.

Moylan J.A., Detmer D.E., Rose J. et al. (1976) Evaluation of quality of hospital care for major trauma. *J. Trauma,* **16,** 517–23.

Nixon J.R. (1976) Late open reduction of traumatic dislocation of the hip. *J. Bone Jt Surg.,* **58B,** 41–3.

Phillips E.H., Rogers W.F. and Gaspar M.R. (1981) First rib fractures: incidence of vascular injury and indications for angiography. *Surgery,* **89,** 42–7.

Preston F.S. and Adicoff A. (1962) Hyperparathyroidism with avulsion of three major tendons. *N. Engl. J. Med.,* **266,** 968–71.

Pringle R.G. (1973) Missed fractures. *Injury,* **4,** 311–6.

Ravichandran G. and Silver J.R. (1982) Missed injuries of the spinal cord. *Br. Med. J.,* **284,** 953–6.

Reid D.C. Henderson R., Saboe L. et al. (1987) Etiology and clinical course of missed spine fractures. *J. Trauma,* **27,** 980–6.

Rose J., Valtonen S. and Jennett B. (1977) Avoidable factors contributing to death after head injury. *Br. Med. J.,* **2,** 615–8.

Sander-Jensen K., Secher N.H., Bie P. et al. (1986) Vagal slowing of the heart during haemorrhage: observations from 20 consecutive hypotensive patients. *Br. Med. J.*, **292**, 364–6.

Shaheen M.A.E.K. and Badr A.A. (1987) Concomitant ipsilateral femoral shaft and femoral neck fracture. *J. R. Coll. Surg. Edinb.*, **32**, 223–7.

Shalley M. and Cross A.B. (1984) Which patients are likely to die in an accident and emergency department? *Br. Med. J.*, **289**, 419–21.

Smith J.T., Keeve J.P., Bertin K.C. et al. (1988) Simultaneous fractures of the distal radius and scaphoid. *J. Trauma*, **28**, 676–9.

Tibbs P.A., Young B., Bivins B.A. et al. (1980) Diagnosis of acute abdominal injuries in patients with spinal shock: value of diagnostic peritoneal lavage. *J. Trauma*, **20**, 55–7.

Trinca G.W. (1982) Diagnostic difficulties in the early management of road crash casualties. In *Care of the acutely ill and injured*. Wilson D.H. and Marsden A.K. (ed.) Chichester, John Wiley, pp. 177–178.

West J.G., Trunkey D.D. and Lim R.C. (1979) Systems of trauma care — a study of two counties. *Arch. Surg.*, **114**, 455–60.

Wilson C.B., Vidrine A. and Rives J.D. (1965) Unrecognised abdominal trauma in patients with head injuries. *Ann. Surg.*, **161**, 608–13.

Yates D.W. (1977) Airway patency in fatal accidents. *Br. Med. J.*, **2**, 1249–51.

23 If you make an error

This chapter should probably be headed 'When you make an error', as the only people who have never misdiagnosed an injury are those who have never treated any. Do not despair therefore for you are not alone in your failings.

As soon as you are aware that you have made a diagnostic error, you should admit this and refer it to someone more senior with experience in dealing with these situations. Never try to cover it up. On occasions the patient may need to be recalled for further investigations or treatment, but many injuries will not need a change of management either because they are minor or because the patient has already been correctly treated. If there has been a delay before the correct diagnosis comes to light, it may be too late for any treatment (e.g. a Colles fracture diagnosed at four weeks or a skull X-ray showing a fracture taking a week to be reported). If the patient is still under review, he should be informed and the problem explained to him and apologized for. Otherwise, all that may be required is a letter to the patient's general practitioner informing him of the missed injury. Failure to inform the GP leaves one open to the accusation of trying to cover it up.

One can learn a lot from one's errors, so obtain the notes and X-rays to work out how the error was made in order to avoid making the same mistake in the future. If it is a missed radiological diagnosis, the X-rays should be presented to a morbidity meeting if this is held, or at least shown to other staff for their education. If it is a 'classical error', copy the X-rays for the departmental X-ray library.

A missed injury may have medicolegal consequences. If this seems likely or if a letter of complaint is received, you may need to inform your defence society who will advise you further. If, on looking at your notes, you realise that your note keeping has been inadequate and that you can remember essential details of the history or examination or of your instructions to the patient which you have not recorded, it is permissible to draw a line under the previous notes and to write down the additional information, using a pen of a different colour and stating that this information was added later on such and such a date.

DO NOT, UNDER ANY CIRCUMSTANCES, TRY TO ALTER THE NOTES YOU MADE AT THE TIME. THIS IS ILLEGAL AND WILL GET YOU INTO VERY BIG TROUBLE.

24 Improving the situation

If errors are to be kept to a minimum, all A & E patients should be seen by well motivated, fully trained doctors working shifts of reasonable length in well staffed departments with good working conditions.

Even if this were to occur, the present junior medical staff might have their working week shortened, but they would still need to be employed, as many other doctors, including general practitioners and surgeons, also treat injured patients and require training. A & E departments also treat patients with medical, surgical, paediatric and other emergencies, and most clinical specialties recognize the value of A & E experience for their trainees.

Increasing the number of fully trained doctors will be expensive (and may not be without other problems) but some savings might be made if trained staff worked faster, ordered fewer investigations, admitted fewer patients and made less errors. Increasing the complement of trained doctors should be aimed for but it will be many years before every patient can expect to be seen by a consultant.

Experience, by itself, is of limited value in improving diagnostic accuracy (Chapter 5) and so it is essential that all doctors employed in A & E and all general practitioners receive appropriate training.

This should start at medical school, where the examination of the musculoskeletal system and the principles of radiological diagnosis should be both taught and formally tested, and the importance of trauma as one of the major causes of mortality and morbidity should be reflected by more emphasis in the curriculum.

All doctors should receive further training in the same subjects *before* starting work in an A & E department, with emphasis being given to commonly missed injuries. A library of X-rays of missed injuries is essential but, for realistic teaching, abnormal X-rays should be presented with normal ones. The general public may feel that they have a right to know that A & E doctors have been formally examined in these skills.

When a doctor starts working, he should initially be supervised and there should always be a more senior doctor in the department to whom he can turn for advice. Formal and informal teaching should continue throughout the appointment, with feedback on specific missed diagnoses and with regular audit of a doctor's performance. Feedback has been shown to improve diagnostic accuracy in abdominal pain (Adams et al., 1986) and so doctors should receive feedback on all their patients and not just their errors. Senior doctors also will benefit from audit, and they too need continuing education, though of a different type from their junior colleagues.

It has been noted earlier in the book that many diagnostic errors have their origin in inadequate history taking and clinical examination. The use of structured forms ensures that all relevant data is collected, and this has been shown to improve diagnostic accuracy of abdominal pain (Adams et al.). In patients with multiple injury the use of such standardized procedures cut the diagnostic error rate in one centre from 23% to 8% (Murat, Huten and Mesny, 1985). The use of proformas for data collection in A & E departments should be investigated and probably expanded.

The use of guidelines has been discussed in Chapter 2. These are useful as long as they are designed with the aim of improving diagnostic accuracy, but not if their intention is to decrease X-ray usage and cut costs. Further research to validate guidelines must be done.

Computer-aided diagnosis has been shown to be more accurate than clinical diagnosis alone for abdominal pain (Adams et al.), not just because of the computer program itself, but also because of the standardized data collection which is necessary and because the computer allows feedback and generates an atmosphere in which junior staff are encouraged to do their best. Most trauma diagnoses in A & E are simple and computer aids are not relevant for most patients who attend, but it should be investigated for certain problems.

X-RAY REPORTING

All doctors examining X-rays will miss a percentage of fractures (hopefully a minimal number with better training) but when X-rays are reviewed by two people they tend to miss different injuries, and so the percentage of injuries missed by both A & E doctor and radiologist is very small (Chapter 3). Therefore, if all X-rays were looked at by an A & E doctor and reported by a consultant radiologist before the patient left the A & E department, the missed diagnosis rate should be dramatically decreased, especially as the radiologist would have the opportunity to ask for more clinical details (which improves his accuracy) (Berbaum et al., 1988) and would also have the opportunity to recommend additional views if there were any doubt. The close links and more teaching should improve the accuracy of A & E doctors too. This must be put forward as an ideal to be aimed at, but its value is not absolutely proven, as the casualty officer may pay less attention to X-rays if they have already been reported or if he knows they will be reported within the next few minutes. Also, as the environment has an effect on diagnostic accuracy (Fowkes, 1986) (Chapter 5) it is also unproven that a radiologist reporting from the hurly burly of a busy A & E department would have the same accuracy as when reporting from a comfortable office.

Even if providing a radiologist for such a 'hot reporting' system were considered too expensive, there are other ways of ensuring that X-rays are looked at by two people.

Over the years, many a disaster has been averted by an experienced radiographer pointing out a fracture, which would otherwise be missed, to an inexperienced doctor, and this informal communication could be formalized. In a study in which both doctors and radiographers (of all grades and without additional training) looked at X-rays separately, the rate of missed diagnoses was almost halved (Berman et al., 1985) (Chapter 3). If radiographers were given specific training for this role, the improvement could be even greater. However, a 'hot reporting' system by radiographers might have similar problems to the potential problems of a 'hot reporting' system by radiologists. There may also be legal problems.

In any system of A & E some injuries will be missed, and it is important that mechanisms exist to pick these up. Most missed diagnoses are injuries missed on X-ray, and so if X-rays are not reported at the time, they should be reported rapidly, and a mechanism should exist whereby the radiologist's report is compared with the casualty officer's diagnosis. If these are found to differ, the casualty officer should be informed (for his own training) and a senior clinician should decide what needs to be done to minimize any harm caused by the missed diagnosis.

FOLLOW-UP CLINICS

Follow-up clinics, such as fracture clinics, are usually organized for the follow-up and management of patients with known injuries, but they are also useful as a long stop to pick up missed injuries. In one series of patients referred to a fracture clinic, 17.2% had had an incorrect diagnosis made in A & E. Most of these were false positives and, of the injuries missed, most had already been correctly treated, but 3.6% of patients had had an injury misdiagnosed and mistreated (Morton, 1988). In another series of patients referred to a hand clinic, 2% had injuries missed (Finlayson et al., 1986). Casualty officers should receive follow-up information on these patients.

It is important that casualty officers be encouraged to send not only known fractures to a follow-up clinic but also any patient whose symptoms and signs are greater than would be expected from the diagnosis.

Lastly, patients should be encouraged to return if their clinical state does not improve. These patients should be seen by senior A &

E staff as, not only will a number of them have had an injury missed, but review of their patients is a useful means of audit.

MULTIPLE INJURIES

The problems of managing the multiply injured patient are numerous and are not just those of diagnosis. Apart from the diagnostic difficulties, these aspects are outside the scope of this book, but essentially patients need early and rapid resuscitation, full diagnosis and early surgery. How this can be achieved is currently the subject of much debate both nationally and internationally (Trunkey, 1985; Royal College of Surgeons, 1988). Most hospitals see relatively few patients with life-threatening injuries and thus cannot provide fully trained and well experienced doctors to be resident 24 hours a day and to have access to an always empty operating theatre for these occasional patients. Experience from the USA indicates that, in centres which treat large numbers of seriously injured patients, diagnostic accuracy (and care in general) is better than in units seeing few patients (West, Trunkey and Lim, 1979).

While debate continues on whether trauma centres are necessary, all hospitals which expect to receive multiply injured patients should organize a system whereby this small but important group of patients can be assessed and managed by experienced doctors (possibly by means of a trauma team) (Spencer, 1985) no matter what the time of the day or night they arrive. The use of protocols and standardized assessment procedures should be encouraged as a means of improving diagnostic accuracy (Murat, Huten and Mesny, 1985).

REFERENCES

Adams I.D., Chan M., Clifford P.C. et al. (1986) Computer aided diagnosis of acute abdominal pain: a multi-centre study. *Br. Med. J.*, **293**, 800–4.
Berbaum K.S., El Khoury G.Y., Franken E.A. et al. (1988) Impact of clinical history on fracture detection with radiography. *Radiology*, **168**, 507–11.

Berman L., de Lacey G., Twomey E. et al. (1985) Reducing errors in the accident department: a simple method using radiographers. *Br. Med. J.*, **290**, 421–2.

Finlayson B.J., Cross A.B., Shalley M.J. et al. (1986) The value of a next day hand injury review clinic. *J. Hand Surg.*, **11B**, 438–40.

Fowkes F.G.R. (1986, Diagnostic vigilance. *Lancet*, **i**, 493–4.

Morton R.S. (1988) Fracture clinic referrals: the need for self audit. *Injury*, **19**, 77–8.

Murat J.E., Huten N. and Mesny J. (1985) The use of standardised assessment procedures in the evaluation of patients with multiple injuries. *Arch. Emerg. Med.*, **2**, 11–5.

Royal College of Surgeons Working Party (1988) The management of patients with major injuries. London, Royal College of Surgeons of England.

Spencer J.D. (1985) Why do our hospitals not make more use of the concept of a trauma team? *Br. Med. J.*, **290**, 136–8.

Trunkey D. (1985) Towards optimal trauma care. *Arch. Emerg. Med.*, **2**, 181–95.

West J.G., Trunkey D.D. and Lim R.C. (1979) Systems of trauma care — a study of two counties. *Arch. Surg.*, **114**, 455–60.

Index

abdominal injury 93–95
   head injury and 174
   spinal injury and 174–5
abscess, wrong diagnosis of 158
abuse *see* non-accidental injury
accessory bones causing confusion on foot
   X-rays 147
accident witnesses 12
acetabulum fracture 127
Achilles tendon rupture 151
   bilateral 178
acromioclavicular joint injuries 100
acromion ossification centre 101
airway obstruction in multiple injuries
   179–80
alcohol intoxication, injury from 46–48
   intracranial haematoma and 66
   spinal 78
alimentary tract foreign body 163–6
aneurysms, false 158
ankle injury 139–48
   avulsion fractures 140, 142
   history taking in 10
   indications for X-ray 139–40
   multiple injuries and 175
   serious fractures 142–3
   tendon injuries, open 153
ankylosing spondylitis, injury and 41
aorta, ruptured 90
arm
   examination in children 46
   flexor tendon rupture 150
   injuries 107–8
   multiple injuries 175–6
   see also elbow; shoulder
artefacts in X-rays causing missed diagnosis
   27

artefactual disease 36
arteries
   injuries 157–8
   in metacarpals appearing as fractures
   123
avulsion fracture of ankle 140, 142

bends in divers 168
biceps tendon avulsion at elbow 107
bilateral injuries 177–8
bladder dysfunction in spinal injury 77
bleeding from ear 67
   mandibular fracture and 83
blood
   loss in multiple injuries 181
   samples for alcohol levels 47–48
blow-out fractures 82
blunt cardiac injuries 89–90
bony injuries
   examination for 14
   normal X-ray and 42–43
boutonnière deformity 150
brachial plexus injuries 153–4
   incorrect diagnosis of 106–7
   spinal injury and 175
brain injury
   alcoholism and 47
   false positive diagnosis of 67–68
breathing problems in multiple injury 180
'buckle fracture' 115
burns 167–8

calcaneum fracture 144–6
cardiac
   injuries, blunt 89–90

193